TABLE OF CONTENTS

Top 20 Test Taking Tips

1. Carefully follow all the test registration procedures
2. Know the test directions, duration, topics, question types, how many questions
3. Setup a flexible study schedule at least 3-4 weeks before test day
4. Study during the time of day you are most alert, relaxed, and stress free
5. Maximize your learning style; visual learner use visual study aids, auditory learner use auditory study aids
6. Focus on your weakest knowledge base
7. Find a study partner to review with and help clarify questions
8. Practice, practice, practice
9. Get a good night's sleep; don't try to cram the night before the test
10. Eat a well balanced meal
11. Know the exact physical location of the testing site; drive the route to the site prior to test day
12. Bring a set of ear plugs; the testing center could be noisy
13. Wear comfortable, loose fitting, layered clothing to the testing center; prepare for it to be either cold or hot during the test
14. Bring at least 2 current forms of ID to the testing center
15. Arrive to the test early; be prepared to wait and be patient
16. Eliminate the obviously wrong answer choices, then guess the first remaining choice
17. Pace yourself; don't rush, but keep working and move on if you get stuck
18. Maintain a positive attitude even if the test is going poorly
19. Keep your first answer unless you are positive it is wrong
20. Check your work, don't make a careless mistake

Theories of Aging

Psychosocial Development

Erik Erikson's Theory of Psychosocial Development describes the development of the personality. According to Erikson, personality develops in eight stages. The first five developmental stages occur in infancy and childhood. The final three stages occur in adulthood. Each stage involves a conflict that must be resolved. Failure to resolve the conflict leads to unhealthy psychosocial development. Resolving the conflict of a particular stage leads to a sense of mastery, while failure to resolve the conflict results in a feeling of inadequacy. Erikson's stages are as follows: trust vs. mistrust (birth to 1 year), autonomy vs. shame/doubt (ages 1 to 3 years); initiative vs. guilt (3 to 6 years), industry vs. inferiority (ages 6 to 12), identity vs. role confusion (ages 12 to 18), intimacy vs. isolation (young adulthood), generativity vs. stagnation (middle age), and ego integrity vs. despair (older adulthood).

Hierarchy of Needs

Abraham Maslow studied individuals he referred to as exemplary people in order to develop his hierarchy of needs. Exemplary people included the likes of Albert Einstein and Eleanor Roosevelt. The top one percent of college students was also included in the group, as these individuals were considered the healthiest in the college population. Maslow felt that studying inferior or unhealthy specimens of humanity could only lead to a crippled theory of psychology. Maslow's Hierarchy of Needs forms a pyramid, with the more basic requirements of life on the bottom of the structure. From top to bottom, these needs are self-actualization, esteem, love/belonging, safety, and physiological. Maslow referred to the needs in the lower four levels as deficiency needs. Deficiency needs must be met first before higher needs can be attended to.

Scott Peck

Scott Peck's Theory of Development proposed four stages. Progression through these stages takes the individual from selfish child to giving elder. The stages are as follows:

- *chaotic/antisocial*: individuals act out of self-interest: they are unprincipled. Babies and children must be taught to act in an ethical and charitable manner.
- *formal/institutional*: individuals want structure. They seek institutions that provide structure. Conformity is an important trait to people in this stage. Individuals may not progress to the third stage.
- *skeptic/individual*: individuals begin to question the rules and beliefs of the institutions they once followed without question. Individuals who do not progress beyond this stage may become depressed and bitter.
- *mystic/communal*: the individual develops a genuine spiritual belief rather than just following the rules. Not all individuals reach this stage.

Theories

Autoimmune Theory

The purpose of the immune system is to protect the body against foreign substances. The Autoimmune Theory of Aging states that the immune system becomes less capable of producing the antibodies to fight disease over time. In addition, the immune system becomes less capable of distinguishing between antibodies produced by the body and proteins. As a result, the body attacks itself. Autoimmune diseases include lupus, rheumatoid arthritis, multiple sclerosis, and scleroderma.

Somatic Mutation Theory

The Somatic Mutation Theory of Aging states that mutations in the cellular DNA lead to dysfunction and disease associated with aging. Although most mutations can be repaired or destroyed, extensive damage to DNA can cause changes in the sequence of genes. The mutated genes copy themselves, leading to disease and diminished functioning. Mutations can occur because of mistakes in cell division. The genes are not copied properly and mutations occur. Mutations can occur as a result of exposure to toxins and radiation.

Social Exchange Theory

Social Exchange Theory is rooted in the following disciplines: structural anthropology, behavioral psychology, utilitarian economics, sociology, and social psychology. The basic tenet of social exchange theory is that an individual interacts with others in the expectation of profit. Each individual acts in a way to reap rewards and avoid punishment and develops a set of strategies to achieve these goals. Behaviors that produce the desired effect are repeated, while those that produce an unwanted effect are not repeated. This learning begins in infancy and continues throughout life. Behaviors and thought processes are, therefore, the result of interactions with society. People in a society are, in effect, trained by other members of society to behave and think in certain ways. George Caspar Homans, an American sociologist, is considered to be the founder of social exchange theory.

Free-Radical Theory

A free radical is any molecule that has unpaired electrons. This creates an unbalanced molecule with a negative charge. As a result of the extra electron, the molecule reacts with balanced molecules in an unhealthy and destructive manner. Constant damage by free radicals will kill a cell. The Free-Radical Theory of Aging proposes that when a large enough number of cells in an organism are killed, aging occurs. Free-radical production in the body can be increased by such things as unhealthy diet, tobacco use, and radiation **exposure.**

Accumulative Waste Theory

The Accumulative Waste Theory of Aging states that cells accumulate more waste products than they can eliminate. The waste products in the cell can include toxins. When the toxins build to a certain level, the cell dies. Aging results when this process occurs in a critical number of cells.

Homeostatic Theory

The human body contains chemical elements in various amounts. The Homeostatic Theory of Aging proposes that aging occurs when the body is unable to maintain proper balance of chemical elements.

Programmed/Cellular Theory

The Programmed/Cellular Theory of Aging states that the life span of every cell and organism is predetermined. Aging occurs as the organism nears the end of the programmed life span.

Single-Organ Theory

The Single-Organ Theory of Aging states that aging results from an alteration in a single vital organ of the body or an alteration in an organ system. For example, it has been suggested that a change in the metabolic rate related to the functioning of the thyroid gland may be responsible for aging. It has also been suggested that aging results from a decreased supply of oxygen.

Stress Theory

The Stress Theory of Aging is described as follows: Any situation or demand (positive or negative) that requires the body to adapt causes stress. The body responds to stress in three physiological stages. The first stage of stress is *alarm*. Alarm causes an increase in the production of adrenaline and cortisol. The release of these chemicals causes the fight-or-flight response. The second stage of the stress response is *resistance*. The body adapts to the new strains or demands. If the stress is not resolved, resistance may become chronic. Long-term stress can lead to organ or system damage. The final stage of the stress response is *exhaustion*. The body can no longer adapt to the stress and is weakened. Organ systems begin to break down at this point, and stress-related diseases occur (for example, gastrointestinal ulcers and atrophy of the thymus gland). Continued stress may lead to death.

Wear-and-Tear Theory

The Wear-and-Tear Theory of Aging posits that the body wears out from use, much like a machine. Over time, damage is done to the cells and systems of the body. Once worn out, the cells and systems cannot repair themselves, and aging occurs. The cells and body systems can no longer function efficiently. This theory has been discredited.

Glycosylation Theory

The Glycosylation Theory of Aging states that aging occurs as a result of the binding of glucose (which is a simple sugar) to protein. This process occurs in the presence of oxygen. The binding of glucose to the protein impairs the actions of the protein. The protein is not able to perform its functions efficiently, and aging results.

Activity

The Activity Theory of Aging states that remaining engaged in life and active has a positive effect on individuals as they age. Older adults can stay active in many ways even if they can't take part in all the activities that they participated in when they were younger. New roles must replace old ones. Staying involved in life has been found to be positively correlated with satisfaction with life.

Disengagement Theory

The Disengagement Theory of Aging was developed by Elaine Cumming and William Henry in 1961. This theory states that to age successfully, an individual should withdraw from society. This disengagement relieves both the aging individual and society from unwanted responsibilities. The withdrawal from society allows the older adult time to reflect and helps keep society functioning smoothly.

Age Stratification/Continuity Theory

The Age Stratification Theory of Aging was developed by Matilda Riley, Marilyn Johnson, and Anne Foner. The theory states that society is divided into age cohorts. The roles of the different cohorts vary, and cohorts differ in status. Individuals in the same age cohort share the same historical context. Individuals born in different eras have had different experiences. For example, individuals who were age 80 in 1950 are not the same as individuals who were age 80 in the year 2000. The events of a particular era affect development, and individuals from the same cohort have shared experiences.

Robert Havighurst, Bernice Neugarten, and Sheldon Tobin postulated that personality type correlates with successful aging. Their Continuity Theory of Aging states that individuals will try to maintain the same lifestyle throughout their lives. Older adults will engage in the same activities and behaviors as they did in their youth. Older adults use strategies to maintain continuity.

Exchange Theory

According to the Exchange Theory Of Aging, interactions between people are based on the exchange of resources. Because older adults often do not have as many resources as younger people, interactions between younger and older individuals are often limited. This occurs because younger adults do not perceive a benefit from interacting with older adults.

Gerotranscendence Theory

The Gerotranscendence Theory Of Aging, formulated by Lars Tornstam, states that older adults experience a cognitive transformation as they age. According to this theory, adults tend to be materialistic when they are younger and become more spiritual as they age. With age comes a focus on external matters and improved relationships. An acceptance of death develops.

Life Course

According to the Life Course Theory of Aging, aging is a process that involves continuing changes from infancy to old age. Changes occur in social, psychological, and biological functioning.

Modernization

Emile Durkheim and Max Weber developed the Modernization Theory of Aging. This theory explains the changing status of older adults in the United States. According to modernization theory, the status of older adults in a society is inversely related to the society's degree of technological development. The status of older adults in a technologically advanced society is lower than in a less technologically advanced society. This is because there are fewer roles that can be filled by older adults in a technologically advanced society.

Person-Environment-Fit

M. Powell Lawton proposed the Person-Environment Fit Theory. This theory states that a person's functional competencies determine how well he or she fits into an environment. Functional competencies include ego strength, motors skills, health, cognitive ability, and sensory-perceptual ability. Functional competencies change with age, and this affects the way people interact with the environment. The loss of functional competencies makes the world a frightening place. This leads to withdrawal from society.

Political Economy Theory

Carroll Estes, James Swan, and Lenore Gerard proposed the Political Economy of Age Theory of Aging. The political and economic requirements of society determine the way older adults are treated. Programs for older adults are designed to serve the needs of society rather than the needs of the older adults.

Role Theory

The Role Theory of Aging was proposed by Irving Rosow. Each person assumes a role in society, which changes with age; each role prepares the individual for the next role. As status is influence by age, role and status may be in conflict. This results in a loss of self-esteem and sense of identity.

Subculture Theory

Rosow also proposed the Subculture Theory of Aging. People in a society form subcultures based on shared interests. Individuals who do not meet inclusion criteria are excluded. Older adults form subcultures based on shared interests and are excluded from the subcultures of younger people. Physical health and mental functioning determine status within the older adult subculture.

Theory of Individualism

Carl Jung proposed, in his Theory of Individualism, that personality continues to develop over an individual's lifetime. Personality is composed of ego, personal unconsciousness, and collective unconsciousness. Although an individual can be introverted or extroverted, emotional health requires a balance between the two. Jung believed that people begin to question their accomplishments, values, and beliefs as they reach middle age. After middle age, people begin to turn inward. Jung believed that successful aging occurs when people value themselves more than they value external factors and when they do not become overly concerned about their physical limitations. Jung believed that it is necessary for an aging adult to accept his or her diminishing capacities in order to age successfully. Older adults must also adapt to change and loss.

Reminiscence Theory

Reminiscence Theory states that reminiscence has benefits for the older adult. There is evidence to suggest that older adults who reminisce are less prone to depression and are mentally healthier than those who don't reminisce. However, the type of reminiscing makes a difference. Idealizing the past or dwelling on negative memories does not have a positive effect. Reminiscence can help the older adult maintain his or her identity.

Self-Efficacy Theory

Self-Efficacy Theory has been applied to aging. It has been suggested that age-related differences in ability may be related to age-related differences in self-efficacy. Older individuals may be unable to perform a function because they believe that they cannot perform this function. This outcome is based on a belief rather than on fact. Higher levels of self-efficacy lead to more successful aging.

Changes

Neurological Changes

Neurological changes associated with aging are detailed here: The number of nerve cells in the brain and spinal cord decreases with increasing age. There is a slight reduction in brain mass. The loss of neurons occurs particularly in the frontal lobes. There is also a decrease in cerebral blood flow. Short-term memory loss may occur with increasing age. Cognitive processes are not usually affected unless there is an underlying brain disease or disorder. For example, Alzheimer's disease and stroke may affect mentation. Some neurofibrillary tangles may be present in the normally aging brain. Skeletal muscles may atrophy with age as a result of peripheral nerve cell degeneration. The ability of peripheral nerves to repair themselves is reduced. The speed of conduction of peripheral nerves may decrease, resulting in a loss of sensation and slower reflexes. There may be changes in the autonomic nervous system, resulting in reduced perspiration.

Cardiovascular Changes

Cardiovascular changes that are associated with aging are listed as follows: There is an age-related reduction in the ability of the cardiovascular system to pump blood. This results in a decrease in oxygen delivery. Reduced cardiac output causes response to situations that call for increased oxygen. The atria may enlarge: This is correlated with atrial fibrillation, atrial flutter, and congestive heart failure (CHF). It should be remembered that there are distinct individual differences in the response of the heart to aging. Some individuals experience much more serious age-related changes than others.circulation

- 9 -

time to increase. Arteries lose elasticity with age, leading to an increase in blood pressure at rest and during exercise. The left ventricle may enlarge (hypertrophy). The baroreceptor response may decrease. Diastolic dysfunction may be evident. An age-related reduction in the resting and maximal heart rates results in a slower

Pulmonary Changes

Pulmonary changes occur with normal aging. There is a decrease in the elasticity of the lungs. The alveoli flatten and the alveolar ducts enlarge. As a result, the air tends to stay in the alveolar ducts rather than in the alveoli. This decreases the efficiency of oxygen exchange. There is an increase in the residual volume of the lungs. There is a reduction in forced expiratory volume (FEV) and forced vital capacity (FVC) in older adults. Because older adults experience a decrease in overall strength, they are less able to breathe deeply. In addition, the cough reflex is reduced. Ciliary action decreases with age. Protective laryngeal reflexes may be lost. Total lung capacity does not change with age.

Skin Changes

The characteristics of the skin change throughout life. The skin of an infant is thinner than that of an adult. The epidermis is fully developed at birth, but the dermis is not and continues to become thicker after birth. During adolescence, the hair follicles in the skin become active, and the dermis becomes thinner. It also takes longer for the cells of the epidermis to regenerate, increasing the time needed for healing. With increasing age, there is a reduction in the number of Langerhans cells. This increases the risk of skin cancer. As the aging process continues, the sweat glands and blood vessels decrease in number, and the amount of subcutaneous fat decreases. This makes the skin drier and more likely to become irritated. The junction between the epidermis and dermis flattens, increasing the risk of tearing. Age and exposure to the sun

break down elastin, which gives skin strength and resilience.

Cognition

There are large individual differences in the effect of age on cognition. Age-related changes in cognition do not usually occur before age 70. Research indicates that approximately 65 percent of individuals exhibit a slight decline in cognitive abilities by age 81. While fluid intelligence (the ability to process information) decreases somewhat, crystallized intelligence (the ability to solve practical problems) is usually unaffected by aging and may actually improve. Acquired knowledge often remains intact. Older adults may find it difficult to apply new information to the solution of complex problems. Even if their intellect is unaffected, older adults may have trouble paying attention for any significant length of time. Individuals older than 60 may take longer to react to situations and may take longer to complete cognitive tasks. Working memory is affected by age. While implicit memory (skills) is unaffected by increasing age, explicit memory (information) may decline.

Basic and Applied Science

Hypertension

Hypertension is commonly called high blood pressure. Blood pressure is defined as the pressure of the blood exerted against the walls of the arteries. An individual's blood pressure results from a combination of cardiac output and peripheral resistance. Hypertension can occur from a change in either one of these factors. Blood pressure is expressed as systolic over diastolic. Normal blood pressure is a systolic pressure less than 120 and a diastolic pressure less than 80. Hypertension is defined as a systolic pressure greater than 140 and a diastolic pressure greater than 90. Primary hypertension is idiopathic, meaning no cause can be identified. Secondary hypertension is defined as hypertension with a known cause (for example, renal disease or thyroid disease). In essential hypertension, cardiac output is within normal limits and peripheral resistance is increased. Hypertension may be caused by an insufficient number of nephrons to adequately clear fluids, stress, genetic anomalies, and obesity.

Hypotension

Hypotension is abnormally low blood pressure. The condition can be life threatening. Low blood pressure is defined as a systolic pressure of 90 mm Hg (millimeters of mercury) or lower and a diastolic pressure of 60 mm Hg or lower. Hypotension can be caused by reduced blood volume (hypovolemia), decreased cardiac output in the presence of normal blood volume, and excessive vasodilation. There are a number of hypotensive syndromes, including orthostatic hypotension, neurocardiogenic syncope, and postprandial hypotension. Orthostatic hypotension is also called postural hypotension. This type of hypotension occurs after following a change the position of the body. Neurocardiogenic syncope occurs as a result of an increase in the activity of the vagus nerve. Postprandial hypotension occurs 30 to 75 minutes after a heavy meal. Orthostatic hypotension and postprandial hypotension occur most commonly in those older than age 65.

Diuretics

A diuretic is any drug that increases the rate of urine formation and urination. This reduces preload. Increasing urine production releases fluids from the body and also reduces salt levels. Diuretics are used to treat peripheral and pulmonary edema, heart failure, some kidney diseases, and hypertension. Diuretics are usually the first medication prescribed for hypertension. Other medications are also prescribed for hypertension to be used in conjunction with diuretics. There are a number of categories of diuretics. These include loop diuretics, thiazide diuretics, and potassium-sparing diuretics. The different categories of diuretics have different mechanisms of action. Diuretics can cause adverse reactions depending on the particular diuretic.

Loop Diuretics

Loop diuretics inhibit the reabsorption of sodium and chloride in the ascending loop of Henle. Loop diuretics also interfere with the reabsorption of magnesium and calcium. Loop diuretics are short acting. Other classes of diuretics many be more appropriate for the treatment of hypertension. Loop diuretics can cause serum levels of potassium, sodium, and magnesium to decrease and calcium levels to increase. This can cause arrhythmia, weakness, and mental confusion. The risk of adverse reactions increases with increasing dosage.

Thiazide Diuretics

Thiazide diuretics act primarily in the distal convoluted tubules and impede the reabsorption of sodium and from the body and an increase in uric acid in the blood. Thiazide diuretics are often given in conjunction with potassium supplements. The effects of thiazide diuretics are long lasting; this class of drug is appropriate for treating hypertension. Side effects include dizziness, postural hypotension, blurred vision, and sun sensitivity.chloride. Thiazide also causes a loss of potassium

Potassium-Sparing Diuretics

Potassium-sparing diuretics act in the late convoluted distal tubules and collecting ducts. This class of drugs inhibits the absorption of sodium but does not promote the secretion of potassium into the urine. Potassium-sparing diuretics cause the kidneys to retain potassium. If administered alone, potassium-sparing diuretics may raise potassium above normal levels. This can cause weakness, arrhythmia, and cardiac arrest. However, because these drugs are not as effective as other diuretics, they are often taken in conjunction with thiazide, which helps to balance potassium levels. Chlorothiazide is a combination of a potassium-sparing diuretic and thiazide. Side effects include dehydration, nausea, insomnia, and blurred vision. Side effects are most likely to occur at the beginning of treatment.

Heart Failure

The Different Classes of Heart Failure

The term heart failure encompasses contraction disorders and/or filling disorders. Contraction disorders involve systolic dysfunction, and filling disorders involve diastolic dysfunction. Heart failure may include pulmonary edema, peripheral edema, or systemic edema. Heart failure has several causes. The most common of these include coronary artery disease, systemic or pulmonary hypertension, cardiomyopathy, abnormal heart valves, and congenital heart disease. Heart failure is classified according to the symptoms involved and the prognosis.

- Class I: Symptoms are not evident during normal activities, and pulmonary congestion and peripheral hypotension are absent. The patient's activities are not restricted. Prognosis is good.
- Class II: Symptoms are usually absent at rest but become evident with physical exertion. Slight pulmonary edema may be present as evidenced by basilar rales. Prognosis is good.
- Class III: Activities of daily living are affected, and the patient experiences discomfort on exertion. Prognosis is fair.
- Class IV: The patient exhibits symptoms at rest. Prognosis is poor.

Acute Heart Failure and Chronic Heart Failure

Acute heart failure can develop within hours or days. It occurs when a functional or structural problem impairs the ability of the heart to pump sufficient blood for the body's needs. The ability of the myocardium to contract decreases. The peripheral blood vessels narrow. Fluid and sodium are retained in an attempt to control hypotension. Heart rate increases. The lack of sufficient oxygen leads to events such as tissue necrosis, cardiotoxicity, pulmonary edema, and organ failure.

Chronic heart failure has a slower development than acute heart failure. The myocardium becomes damaged by insufficient oxygenation and nutrition. Myocardial cells die, and areas of the heart become necrotic. Fibroblasts are produced in response, and dead myocardial cells are replaced with collagen. This process results in a fibrotic heart muscle. Existing myocardial cells enlarge and become weaker. Cardiac dilation and vascular resistance are the end results.

Systolic Heart Failure

Systolic heart failure is left-sided heart failure. This type of heart failure decreases the volume of blood pumped from the ventricles during each contraction. The sympathetic nervous system produces epinephrine and norepinephrine to support the heart muscle. Down-regulation eventually results, and the beta and adrenergic receptors are destroyed. This causes further damage to the heart muscle. The reduced perfusion stimulates the kidneys to produce rennin. This promotes the release of angiotensin I, which is converted to angiotensin II. Angiotensin II is a vasoconstrictor. This stimulates the production of aldosterone, which causes sodium and fluid to be retained. Preload and afterload are increased as a result of these processes, adding to the workload of the heart. The myocardium loses its ability to contract, and blood accumulates in the ventricles. The myocardium is stretched, and the ventricles enlarge. The heart muscle thickens, and ischemia results due to an insufficient blood supply.

Diastolic Heart Failure

The clinical symptoms of diastolic heart failure and systolic heart failure are similar. In diastolic heart failure, the heart muscle cannot relax sufficiently to allow the ventricles to fill. This is similar to what occurs in systolic heart failure, when myocardial hypertrophy causes stiffening of the muscle. Diastolic heart failure occurs more commonly in women older than 75 years of age. In diastolic heart failure, the intracardiac pressure is usually within the normal range. However, the pressure increases substantially on exertion. The ventricles of the heart do not expand adequately for the fill volume, and the heart is unable to increase stroke volume during exercise because of the delay in muscle relaxation. Dyspnea, fatigue, and pulmonary edema are evident on exercise as a result. Ejection fractions are generally greater than 40 or 50 percent. There is a rise in left ventricular end-diastolic pressure (LVEDP). Left ventricular end-diastolic volume (LVEDV) decreases.

Myocardial Infarction

Myocardial infarction (MI) results when the supply of oxygen to the heart is not sufficient to meet its requirements. MI is on the acute coronary syndrome (ACS) continuum. An MI may result after any of the following events: an episode of unstable angina resulting from rupture of an atherosclerotic plaque, thrombosis associated with coronary artery spasm, vasoconstriction, acute blood loss, a reduction in the oxygen supply, and cocaine ingestion. Myocardial damage usually occurs in the following stages: 1) ischemia develops with decreasing oxygen levels, resulting in an ischemic zone; 2) cellular damage occurs to the cells surrounding the site of infarction; and 3) tissue becomes necrotic at the site of infarction, and the cells are replaced with scar tissue. A myocardial infarction (MI) is categorized according to the extent of the damage and necrosis, the location of the damage, and the muscle layers affected.

The Clinical Manifestations of MI

The clinical manifestations of MI vary considerably among individuals. Males usually exhibit the more classical symptoms of MI. Females often do not exhibit these symptoms. Patients with diabetes may have reduced pain sensation because of neuropathy. A diabetic patient with MI may complain primarily of weakness. Elderly patients may also have a reduced sensation of pain and complain of weakness during MI. Older individuals with MI are more likely to exhibit pulmonary edema, left ventricular wall rupture, or papillary muscle rupture.

Signs and symptoms of MI include chest pain (66%), dyspnea (20–59%), neurological symptoms (15–33%), and gastrointestinal tract disorders (20%). Other signs and symptoms may include hypertension and hypotension. Electrocardiogram (ECG) changes may be evident (arrhythmia, tachycardia, bradycardia, or dysrhythmia).

Pharmacologic Measures Taken to Maximize Perfusion

The purpose of using <u>pharmacologic measures</u> to maximize <u>perfusion</u> is to reduce the risk of thrombosis.

- Antiplatelet drugs (for example, aspirin, Ticlid, and Plavix) inhibit clotting by interfering with the plasma membrane function. These drugs prevent the formation of clots but are ineffective at treating existing clots.
- Vasodilators help divert blood away from areas of ischemia. Some of these drugs, such as Pietal, dilate arteries and reduce clotting. Pietal is administered to control intermittent claudication.
- Antilipemics (for example, Zocor and Questran) slow the progression of atherosclerosis.
- Hemorheologics (such as Trental) decrease fibrinogen. This reduces blood viscosity and erythrocyte rigidity. These drugs may be used to treat intermittent claudication.
- Analgesics may be used to improve the quality of life. *Opioids* may be needed for severe pain.
- Thrombolytics (for example, streptokinase) may be administered to dissolve clots. The drug is injected into a blocked artery under angiography.
- Anticoagulants (such as Coumadin and Lovenox) prevent the formation of blood clots.

Digitalis Drugs

Digitalis drugs, the most common of which is digoxin (Lanoxin), are made from the foxglove plant. These drugs are administered to increase contractility of the heart muscle, increase left ventricular output, and slow conduction through the atrioventricular (AV) node. The drug lowers a rapid heart rate and promotes diuresis. Although digoxin does not decrease the incidence of death, it does increase activity tolerance and reduce the number of hospitalizations for heart failure. It is essential not to exceed therapeutic levels (0.5–2.0 ng/mL) in order to avoid toxicity. Toxicity can occur even if therapeutic levels are not exceeded. Early signs and symptoms of toxicity include increasing fatigue, depression, nausea, and vomiting. Later symptoms include sudden changes in heart rhythm, sinoatrial (SA) or AV block, dysrhythmia, and tachycardia. Digitalis toxicity is treated by discontinuation of the medication and serum monitoring. Digoxin immune FAB (Digibind) may be administered to inactivate digoxin.

ACE Inhibitors/Beta-Blockers/Aldosterone Agonists

A number of different types of medication are used to treat heart failure and hypertension.

- ACE inhibitors, such as captopril (Capoten), enalapril (Vasotec), and lisinopril (Prinivil), reduce afterload and preload and reverse ventricular remodeling. However, they may initially cause hypotension and are contraindicated for individuals with renal insufficiency.
- Beta-blockers, such as metoprolol (Lopressor), carvedilol (Coreg), and esmolol (Brevibloc), decrease the heart rate, reduce hypertension, prevent dysrhythmia, and reverse ventricular remodeling. However, these drugs should not be used during decompensation. Individuals with airway disease, uncontrolled diabetes,

a slow/irregular pulse, or heart block should be monitored carefully while taking beta-blockers.

- Aldosterone agonists, such as spironolactone (Aldactone), reduce preload, myocardial hypertrophy, and edema. These drugs may increase blood levels of potassium.

Smooth-Muscle Relaxants

Smooth-muscle relaxants (vasodilators) improve heart function by dilating the arteries or veins. These agents may be administered as a treatment for pulmonary hypertension or generalized systemic hypertension. Vasodilators may be taken by individuals who cannot tolerate angiotensin-converting enzyme (ACE) inhibitors or angiotensin-receptor blockers. Dilation of arteries reduces afterload and improves cardiac output. Dilation of veins reduces preload, decreasing filling pressures. Smooth-muscle relaxants reduce peripheral vascular resistance. However, they may cause hypotension and headaches.

There are a number of types of vasodilators:

- Sodium nitroprusside (Nipride) dilates arteries and veins. This agent is used to reduce hypertension and afterload for heart failure. It has a fast onset of action.
- Nitroglycerin (Tridil) dilates veins primarily and is administered intravenously to reduce preload in acute heart failure, unstable angina, and acute myocardial infarction (MI). Nitroglycerin may also be administered after percutaneous coronary intervention (PCI) to prevent vasospasm.
- Hydralazine (Apresoline) dilates arteries. This drug is administered intermittently in the treatment of hypertension.

Calcium Channel Blockers

Calcium channel blockers are primarily arterial vasodilators. These agents may cause dilation of the peripheral and/or coronary arteries. Side effects include fatigue, flushing, abdominal and peripheral edema, and indigestion.

- Dihydropyridines, such as nifedipine (Procardia) and nicardipine (Cardene), are primarily arterial vasodilators. These drugs dilate both coronary and peripheral arteries and are administered in the treatment of acute hypertension.
- Benzothiazines, such as diltiazem (Cardizem), and phenylalkylamines, such as verapamil (Calan, Isoptin), dilate coronary arteries primarily. These agents are used to treat angina and supraventricular tachycardia.
- ACE inhibitors cause vasodilation by limiting the production of angiotensin. These drugs may cause a large drop in blood pressure, so individuals taking ACE inhibitors must be carefully monitored. These are first-line agents in the treatment of acute hypertension and heart failure and are also administered to prevent nephropathy in patients with diabetes.

Captopril (Capoten) and *enalapril* (Vasotec) are administered to reduce afterload and preload in cases of heart failure.

B-Type Natriuretic Peptides, Alpha-Adrenergic Blockers, and Selective Specific Dopamine DA1-Receptor Agonists

B-type natriuretic peptide (BNP), available as nesiritide (Natrecor), is a new kind of vasodilator. BNP is a recombinant form of a peptide found in the human brain. BNP reduces filling pressure and vascular resistance. It increases the output of urine. BNP may cause hypotension, headache, bradycardia, and nausea.

Alpha-adrenergic blockers cause vasodilation of arteries and veins by blocking alpha receptors. Side effects include orthostatic hypotension and edema from fluid retention. Labetalol (Normodyne) is a combination drug. It is a peripheral alpha-blocker and cardiac beta-blocker. This drug is used in the treatment of acute hypertension, acute stroke, and acute aortic dissection. Phentolamine (Regitine) dilates the peripheral arteries. It reduces afterload and is used to treat pheochromocytoma. Selective specific dopamine DA1-receptor agonists, such as fenoldopam (Corlopam), are peripheral dilators. They dilate renal and mesenteric arteries. These drugs can be used to treat renal dysfunction. They can also be used to treat individuals at risk for renal insufficiency.

PAD

Peripheral vascular insufficiency is inadequate peripheral blood flow. It can involve both veins and arteries. Peripheral venous insufficiency is a chronic disorder and does not usually cause crises requiring acute care. Peripheral arterial disease (PAD) affects the aorta, arteries, and arterioles. In PAD, the arteries of the legs are often occluded. This causes extreme pain and ischemia. The distal aorta and femoral, popliteal, and iliac arteries are the vessels most commonly affected by peripheral arterial disease. Atherosclerosis is the most frequent cause of peripheral disease. Symptoms of PAD include intermittent claudication (cramping pain while walking), rest pain, and tissue changes (thickening of the nails, hair loss, dry skin, and ulcerations). These symptoms require treatment to remove the blockage (catheter or surgery). Acute occlusion may present with pain, lack of pulses, reduced skin temperature, reduced sensation, and loss of function. Acute occlusion requires immediate surgical intervention.

Coronary Artery Disease

Coronary (arteriosclerotic) artery disease (CAD) is the most frequently occurring cardiovascular disorder. Increased high-density lipoprotein (HDL) cholesterol levels initiate an inflammatory process, which damages the arterial lining. Low-density lipoprotein (LDL) cholesterol and monocytes then enter the tissue. A percentage of the monocytes turn into macrophages. The macrophages in combination with LDL cholesterol form foam cells. Foam cells are an indicator of atherosclerosis. HDL aids in clearing cholesterol from the lining of the artery. Plaques with a procoagulant lipid center and fibrous cap develop. If the cap ruptures, the lipids are released and may block the lumen. This can result in a thrombosis and lead to myocardial infarction if there is insufficient collateral circulation. Plaques may decrease in size with a decrease in serum cholesterol level. In this case, the lipid core shrinks and inflammation decreases. However, the fibrous cap of the plaque remains intact. HDL may be raised and LDL lowered by medications and changes in diet.

Dysrhythmias

Cardiac dysrhythmias are abnormal heart rhythms. They often occur as a result of damage to the conduction system. Damage may occur during major cardiac surgery or after a myocardial infarction.

Bradydysrhythmias involve abnormally slow pulse rates.

Complete atrioventricular (AV) block may be congenital or occur as a response to surgical trauma.

Sinus bradycardia may be caused by the autonomic nervous system or occur because of hypotension and a decrease in available oxygen.

Junctional/nodal rhythms occur frequently in postsurgical patients when the P wave is absent. Heart rate and output generally remain stable. Unless there is compromise, no treatment is necessary.

Tachydysrhythmias are abnormally fast pulse rates.

Sinus tachycardia is often caused by illness.

Supraventricular tachycardia (200–300 beat per minute) often has a sudden onset and leads to congestive heart failure.

Conduction irregularities are irregular heart rhythms that occur postoperatively. They are usually of no significance.

Premature contractions originate in the atria or ventricles.

Sinus Node Dysrhythmias

Sinus arrhythmia (SA) originates in the sinus node. The arrhythmia is often paradoxical, which means it increases with inspiration and decreases with expiration. This occurs because the vagal nerve is stimulated during inspiration. A negative hemodynamic effect rarely occurs as a result of sinus arrhythmia. Cyclical changes often occur in the pulse during respiration in both children and young adults. These changes often decrease with age. In some adults, they may persist. In some cases, sinus arrhythmia is associated with heart or valvular disease. Vagal stimulation that occurs during suctioning, vomiting, or defecating may increase sinus arrhythmia.

Sinus bradycardia (SB) results from a decreased impulse rate from the sinus node. The pulse and electrocardiogram (ECG) are abnormally slow but otherwise normal. SB is characterized by a regular heart rhythm with a pulse rate of fewer than 60 beats per minute (bpm). P waves are in front of QRS waves, which are generally normal in shape and duration. The PR interval is 0.12–0.20

seconds, and the P:QRS ratio is 1:1. There are a number of factors that can cause SB:

- Conditions that reduce the body's metabolic requirements (for example, hypothermia or sleep)
- Some medications (such as calcium channel blockers and beta-blockers)
- Vagal stimulation resulting from vomiting, suctioning, or defecating
- Increased intracranial pressure
- Myocardial infarction.

SB is treated by eliminating the cause of the disorder (for example, changing medications). Atropine 0.5–1.0 mg may be administered intravenously to block vagal stimulation.

Sinus tachycardia (ST) occurs as a result of an increase in the frequency of the sinus node impulse. ST is characterized by a regular pulse greater than 100 bpm. P waves occur before the QRS waves but are sometimes part of the preceding T wave. The shape and duration of the QRS waves are usually normal, but they may be consistently irregular. The PR interval is 0.12–0.20 seconds, and the P:QRS ratio is 1:1. The rapid pulse results in a decrease in the diastolic filling time and a reduction in cardiac output, resulting in hypotension. Decreased ventricular filling may lead to acute pulmonary edema. A number of factors may cause ST:

- Acute blood loss
- Shock
- Anemia
- Hypovolemia
- Sinus arrhythmia
- Heart failure (hypovolemic)
- Hypermetabolic conditions
- Fever
- Anxiety
- Exertion
- Medications (such as sympathomimetic drugs).

Treatment for ST includes eliminating the precipitating factors and reducing heart rate by means of calcium channel blockers and beta-blockers.

Atrial Dysrhythmias

A premature atrial contraction (PAC) is an extra beat caused by an electrical impulse to the atrium occurring before the sinus node impulse. This occurrence may be the result of alcohol, caffeine, or nicotine intake. PACs may also occur as a result of hypervolemia, hypokalemia, hypermetabolic conditions, atrial ischemia, or infarction. There is an irregular pulse because of extra P waves. Although the shape and duration of the QRS wave is usually normal, it may be abnormal. The PR interval is between 0.12–0.20 seconds. The P:QRS ratio is 1:1. PACs can occur in healthy hearts and are not cause for concern unless they occur at a rate of more than six per hour and cause severe palpitations. In severe cases, atrial fibrillation may be the cause and antidysrhythmic drugs may be required. Eliminating the cause usually helps to control the PACs.Atrial flutter (AF) results from an atrial rate that is faster (250–400 beats per minute [bpm]) than the conduction rate of the atrioventricular (AV) node. Not all of the impulses continue through into the ventricles. The impulses are blocked at the AV node. AF is caused by coronary artery disease, valvular disease, pulmonary disease, heavy alcohol ingestion, and cardiac surgery. Atrial rates reach 250–400, while ventricular rates reach 75–150; the ventricular rate is generally regular. The P waves are saw-toothed. These are referred to as fibrillatory (F) waves. The shape and duration of QRS waves are usually normal. It is difficult to calculate the PR interval because of F waves. The P:QRS ratio is 2:1–4:1. Symptoms include chest pain, dyspnea, and hypotension. There are a number of treatments for atrial fibrillation. Cardioversion is performed if the condition is unstable. Medications may be administered to control the heart rate. Medications may also be given to cause conversion to sinus rhythm.Atrial fibrillation (A Fib) involves rapid, disorganized atrial beats. A Fib can cause the formation of thrombus and emboli. The ventricular rate increases, while the stroke volume decreases. Cardiac output decreases, and myocardial ischemia increases. There are a number of causes for A Fib, including coronary artery disease, valvular disease, pulmonary disease, heavy alcohol ingestion, and cardiac surgery. In A Fib, the pulse is very irregular; the atrial rate is 300–600 bpm, and the ventricular rate is 120–200 bpm. Generally, the shape and duration of QRS waves are normal. Instead of P waves, fibrillatory (F) waves are seen. It is impossible to measure the PR interval. The P:QRS ratio varies. Cardioversion may be required if A Fib lasts longer than 48 hours. However, the condition frequently converts to normal sinus rhythm within 24 hours. There are a number of medications administered to treat A Fib. Ibutilide, procainamide, and digoxin are used to treat acute A Fib. Quinidine and amiodarone are administered to maintain rhythm. Ventricular rate is controlled by means of beta-blockers, calcium channel blockers, and verapamil. Heparin and Coumadin are given to prevent clotting.

Ventricular Dysrhythmias

In a premature ventricular contraction (PVC) the electrical impulse starts in the ventricles and continues through the ventricles before the next sinus impulse. There may be one site (unifocal) or multiple sites (multifocal) stimulating the ectopic beats. For this reason, QRS complexes vary in shape. Unless there is an underlying heart condition or an acute myocardial infarction (MI), PVCs do not usually cause death. Characteristics of PVCs include an irregular heartbeat, an oddly shaped QRS wave that is greater than or equal to 0.12 seconds, an absent P wave or a P wave that precedes or follows the QRS wave, a PR interval of less than 0.12 seconds in cases in which a P wave is present, and a P:QRS ratio of 0:1–1:1. PVCs are often left untreated in healthy individuals, but lidocaine may be administered as a short-term treatment. PVCs may be triggered by caffeine, nicotine, or alcohol. PVCs may occur in conjunction with any type of supraventricular dysrhythmia, so the underlying rhythm must be determined as well.

Ventricular tachycardia (VT) is defined as three or more PVCs in sequence with a ventricular rate of 100–200 bpm. Ventricular tachycardia and PVCs may have the same triggers, and both may be related to underlying coronary artery disease. However, the rapid rate of contractions during VT makes the condition dangerous. The heart does not pump blood efficiently during VT, and the ineffective beats may cause unconsciousness. If a rate is detectable, it is usually regular. The oddly shaped QRS complex is greater than or equal to 0.12 seconds. The P wave may or may not be present. If the P wave is present, the PR interval is irregular. The P:QRS ratio may be difficult to detect because of the absence of P waves. Treatment varies, depending on the severity of the condition. It may be necessary to use cardioversion to restore a normal sinus rhythm, but ventricular tachycardia (VT) may convert spontaneously. If the patient is unconscious and no pulse can be felt, defibrillation is usually administered as an emergency measure.

Ventricular fibrillation (VF) is a rapid and very irregular ventricular rate. The ventricles beat at more than 300 beats per minute (bpm), but no atrial activity is observable on the electrocardiogram (ECG). The condition results from disorganized electrical activity in the ventricles. The QRS complex is not discernable; the ECG shows irregular undulations. The causes of ventricular fibrillation are the same as for ventricular tachycardia (VT). These include alcohol, caffeine, and nicotine intake and underlying coronary disease. If VT is left untreated, VF may result. Electrical shock can induce VF.

Congenital disorders, such as Brugada syndrome, can also cause VF. Individuals with VF do not have a palpable pulse or audible pulse and lack respirations. VF is a life-threatening condition, and emergency defibrillation is necessary. The cause of the condition should be determined after normal rhythm is established. Antiarrhythmic agents (such as amiodarone) may be alternated with defibrillation to convert the heart rhythm to normal rhythm. If VF occurs as a result of MI, the mortality rate is high.

Classified/Unclassified Antidysrhythmics

Antidysrhythmics are drugs that control dysrhythmia by acting on the conduction system, the ventricles, and/or the atria. There are four classes of antidysrhythmic drugs and some unclassified antidysrhythmics:

- Class I includes three subtypes of sodium channel blockers (quinidine, lidocaine, and procainamide).
- Class II includes beta-blockers (esmolol and propranolol).
- Class III drugs slow repolarization (amiodarone and ibutilide).
- Class IV includes calcium channel blockers (diltiazem and verapamil).
- Unclassified drugs include adenosine. Different drugs are used for specific dysrhythmias. Antidysrhythmic drugs are used to treat paroxysmal supraventricular tachycardia, atrial fibrillation, atrial flutter, sinus tachycardia, PVCs, ventricular tachycardia, and ventricular fibrillation. All of these drugs have specific uses and are associated with adverse effects.

Adverse Side Effects

Adenosine is used to terminate episodes of supraventricular tachycardia. The drug acts to cause a transient heart block at the atrioventricular (AV) node. Adenosine is also a vasodilator. Side effects include facial flushing, asystole, excessive sweating, and light-headedness.

Amiodarone (Cordarone) acts on the atria and ventricles and may cause a reduction in blood pressure (BP) and have adverse effects on the liver.

Digoxin (Lanoxin) acts on the conduction system. It decreases the conduction rate through the AV node. It increases the force at which the heart muscles contract. It may cause bradycardia, heart block, nausea and vomiting, and central nervous system (CNS) depression.

Diltiazem (Cardizem, Tiazac) decreases conduction through the AV node and may cause arrhythmia, bradycardia, and palpitations.

Ibutilide (Corvert) acts on the conduction system. It can cause a severe and potentially fatal arrhythmia called polymorphic ventricular tachycardia. Although this usually occurs in conjunction with QT prolongation, this is not always the case.

Esmolol (Brevibloc) acts on the conduction system and may cause a reduction in BP, bradycardia, and heart failure.

Lidocaine acts on the ventricles and may cause CNS toxicity, nausea, and vomiting.

Procainamide affects the atria and ventricles of the heart. Use of this drug may result in a reduction in BP and electrocardiogram (ECG) abnormalities (widening of QRS and QT).

Verapamil (Calan, Verelan) acts on the conduction system and may cause a reduction in BP, bradycardia, and heart failure.

Specific Dysrhythmia Drugs

Supraventricular tachycardia is treated with diltiazem (Cardizem and Tiazac), esmolol (Brevibloc), propranolol (Inderal), and procainamide.

Paroxysmal supraventricular tachycardia is treated with adenosine, digoxin (Lanoxin), and verapamil (Calan, Verelan).

Atrial fibrillation is treated with digoxin (Lanoxin), diltiazem (Cardizem and Tiazac), ibutilide (Corvert), and amiodarone (Cordarone).

Atrial flutter is treated with digoxin (Lanoxin), diltiazem (Cardizem and Tiazac), ibutilide (Corvert), verapamil (Calan and Verelan), amiodarone (Cordarone), and procainamide.

Sinus tachycardia is treated with esmolol (Brevibloc).

Premature ventricular contractions are treated with lidocaine and procainamide.

Ventricular tachycardia is treated with lidocaine, amiodarone (Cardizem, Tiazac), and procainamide.

Ventricular fibrillation is treated with lidocaine.

First-Degree AV Block

First-degree atrioventricular (AV) block describes a situation in which the atrial impulses are conducted through the AV node to the ventricles at a slower-than-normal rate. The P waves and QRS complex are usually normal. The PR interval is greater than 0.20 seconds, and the P:QRS ration is 1:1. If the QRS complex is narrow, it indicates that the conduction abnormality is only in the AV node. A widened QRS complex indicates that the bundle branches are also damaged. Chronic first-degree AV block may result from the fibrosis/sclerosis associated with coronary artery disease, valvular disease, and cardiac myopathies. This type of block is not usually associated with morbidity. Acute first-degree block is potentially much more serious and may occur as a result of digoxin toxicity, beta-blockers, amiodarone, myocardial infarction, hyperkalemia, or edema resulting from valvular surgery. The condition is correlated with increasing age. The incidence of first-degree AV block is low in young adults. However, elderly individuals have a lower rate of first-degree AV block (at 5%) than do athletes (8.7%).

Second-Degree AV Blocks

Second-degree AV block describes a situation in which some of the atrial beats are blocked at the AV node. Second-degree AV block is divided into two types based on the pattern of blockage:

Mobitz type I block (Wenckebach): In type I block, the interval between the atrial impulses in a group of beats increases until one fails to conduct (the PR interval progressively increases). This results in more P waves than QRS waves. However, the shape and duration of the QRS complex is usually normal. The sinus node conducts impulses at a regular rate, so the P-P interval is regular. However, the R-R interval usually becomes shorter with each impulse. The P:QRS ratio varies (for example, 3:2, 4:3, or 5:4). This type of block does not usually cause significant morbidity unless it is associated with inferior-wall myocardial infarction. If this occurs, a temporary pacemaker may be needed.

In Mobitz type II block, some of the atrial impulses are conducted unpredictably through the AV node to the ventricles. The block always occurs below the AV node in the bundle of His, the bundle branches, or the Purkinje fibers. If the impulses are conducted, the PR intervals do not vary. In most cases, the QRS complex is widened. The P:QRS ratio varies (for example, 2:1, 3:1, and 4:1). Type II block is more serious than type I block. Type II block progress to complete AV block and may cause Stokes-Adams syncope. In addition, if the block occurs at the Purkinje fibers, there is no escape impulse. In the case of type II block, a transcutaneous cardiac pacemaker and defibrillator should be kept at the patient's bedside. If the heart block is caused by myocarditis or myocardial ischemia, chest pain may be experienced.

In a 2:1 block, every other atrial impulse (P:QRS ratio of 2.1) is conducted through the AV node. A 2:1 block may be referred to as advanced second-degree AV block.

Third-Degree AV Block

In third-degree AV block, the P waves outnumber the QRS waves and there is no clear relationship between the two. The atrial rate is 2–3 times the speed of the pulse rate. Because of this, the PR interval is irregular. In the case of sinoatrial (SA) node malfunction, the AV node fires at a lower rate. In the case of AV node malfunction, the pacemaker site in the ventricles takes over, resulting in a bradycardic rate. If there is a complete AV block, the heart still contracts. However, the contractions are often ineffectual. Atrioventricular dissociation occurs because the atrial P wave (sinus rhythm or atrial fibrillation) and the ventricular QRS wave (ventricular escape rhythm) are stimulated by different impulses. While the heart may be able to compensate at rest, it cannot compensate when placed under stress (exertion). Bradycardia results and may lead to congestive heart failure, syncope (fainting), or sudden death. Conduction abnormalities usually worsen gradually over time. Symptoms include dyspnea (shortness of breath), chest pain, and hypotension. Atropine is administered intravenously for these symptoms. The use of a transcutaneous pacemaker may be required. Complete persistent atrioventricular (AV) block normally requires an implanted pacemaker, usually dual chamber.

COPD

Chronic obstructive lung disease (COPD) includes emphysema and chronic bronchitis. These disorders may occur separately or in combination. COPD causes a progressive limitation in airflow. The disease process includes an inflammatory response that results in a narrowing of the peripheral airways and thickening of the pulmonary blood vessel walls. Symptoms include chronic cough, dyspnea, and orthopnea. Acute episodes can result in decompensation with hypoxemia (arterial oxygen saturation [SAO_2] greater than 90 with tachycardia, tachypnea, cyanosis, and change in mental status) and hypercapnia (mental status change and hypopnea). Assessment for severity includes pulmonary function tests, arterial blood gas (ABG) level, chest x-ray (to rule out pneumonia or other complications), and echocardiogram. Treatments include oxygen with nasal cannula, face mask, Venturi mask, or nonrebreathing mask to elevate partial pressure of oxygen in arterial blood (PAO_2) to greater than 60 mm Hg or SAO_2 to greater than 90 percent; beta-2 adrenergic agonists by nebulizer for bronchodilation; anticholinergics (ipratropium bromide by metered inhaler); corticosteroids (60–180 mg/day for 7–14 days in decreasing doses); antibiotics for infection; and assisted ventilation for muscle fatigue and respiratory acidosis.

Chronic Bronchitis

Chronic bronchitis is a pulmonary airway disease defined by severe cough with sputum production lasting at least two years. Irritation of the airways causes an inflammatory response that increases the number of mucus-secreting glands and goblet cells. Ciliary function also decreases, allowing the extra mucus to plug the airways. In addition, the bronchial walls become thicker, and alveoli near the inflamed bronchioles become fibrotic. These changes prevent the alveolar macrophages from functioning properly. As a result, susceptibility to infection is increased. Chronic bronchitis occurs most frequently in individuals older than age 45. It occurs twice as often in females than in males. Symptoms include persistent cough with increasing amounts of sputum, dyspnea, and frequent respiratory tract infections. Treatment for chronic bronchitis includes bronchodilators, long-term continuous oxygen therapy, supplemental oxygen during exercise as required, pulmonary rehabilitation to improve exercise and breathing, antibiotics for infection, and corticosteroids for acute episodes.

Emphysema

Emphysema involves abnormal enlargement of air spaces at the ends of terminal bronchioles and destruction of the alveolar walls. As a result, gas exchange decreases and dead space increases. These changes lead to hypoxemia, hypercapnia, and respiratory acidosis. The capillary bed is damaged, resulting in an increased pulmonary blood flow and raised pressure in the right atrium (cor pulmonale) and pulmonary artery. Cardiac failure results from these changes. Complications of emphysema include respiratory insufficiency and failure. The two primary types of emphysema are centrilobular and panlobular. These may occur together. *Centrilobular* is the most common type. It affects the central portion of the respiratory lobule, sparing distal alveoli and usually the upper lobes. Symptoms include abnormal ventilation-perfusion ratios, hypoxemia, hypercapnia, and polycythemia with right-sided heart failure. *Panlobular* emphysema is an enlargement of all air spaces, including the bronchiole, alveolar duct, and alveoli. However, there is minimal inflammatory disease. Symptoms include hyperextended, rigid, barrel chest; marked dyspnea; weight loss; and active expiration.

Aspiration Pneumonitis and Pneumonia

Aspiration pneumonitis and pneumonia result from the inhalation of toxic substances (for example, stomach contents). The inhaled substance damages the lungs. The risk factors for aspiration pneumonitis and pneumonia include an altered level of consciousness related to illness or sedation, certain diseases (such as Alzheimer's and Parkinson's), depression of the gag or swallowing reflex, intubation or feeding tubes, ileus or gastric distention, and gastrointestinal disorders (for example, gastroesophageal reflux disorders). Diagnosis is based on clinical findings, arterial blood gases showing hypoxemia, infiltrates observed on x-ray and an increased white blood cell count if infection is present. Symptoms are similar to other pneumonias and include cough (often with copious sputum), dyspnea, respiratory distress, cyanosis, tachycardia, and hypotension. Treatment includes suctioning as needed to clear the upper airway, supplemental oxygen, antibiotic therapy as indicated, and symptomatic respiratory support.

Pneumonia

Pneumonia is an inflammation of the lung parenchyma; the alveoli fill with exudate. Pneumonia is a common disease, occurring in children and adults. Pneumonia may be a primary or secondary disease. It may occur as a result of another infection or disease. Pneumonia may be caused by bacteria, viruses, parasites, or fungi. There are a number of common causes for community-acquired pneumonia: *Streptococcus pneumoniae*, legionella species, *Haemophilus influenzae*, *Staphylococcus aureus*, *Mycoplasma pneumoniae*, and viruses.

Chemical damage may also cause pneumonia. Pneumonia is categorized according to site of infection. *Lobar pneumonia* involves one or more lobes of the lungs. If the pneumonia involves lobes in both lungs, it is referred to as bilateral or double pneumonia.

Bronchial/lobular pneumonia involves the terminal bronchioles, and *exudate pneumonia* can involve the adjacent lobules. The pneumonia usually occurs in scattered patches throughout the lungs. *Interstitial pneumonia* primarily affects the interstitium and alveoli. White blood cells and plasma fill the alveoli, causing inflammation and creating fibrotic tissue as the alveoli are destroyed.

Lung Cancer

Lung cancer is the leading cause of cancer-related death in adults older than age 65. Approximately 80 to 90 percent of lung cancer is related to a history of smoking. Four types of lung cancer occur commonly in older adults:

- Squamous cell cancer (40–50%) affects the central airway and is slow growing.
- Adenocarcinoma (30–35%) affects the bronchial/mucosal glands and is more lethal than squamous cell cancer.
- Large-cell cancer (15%) affects the bronchial/mucosal glands.
- Small-cell (oat-cell) cancer (25%) affects the submucosal tissue, grows rapidly, and metastasizes rapidly (often by the time of diagnosis).

Symptoms depend on whether the cancer is localized or has spread. Symptoms can include cough, respiratory obstruction, pain, dyspnea, hoarseness, superior vena cava syndrome pneumonitis, pleural effusion, dysphagia, bronchoesophageal fistula, arrhythmia, and heart failure. Initial diagnosis is based on x-ray and computed tomography (CT). However, false negatives can occur. Cytologic screening may not detect cancer in the early stages. Treatment depends on the stage of the cancer and may include chemotherapy, surgery, or palliative care.

Tuberculosis

Tuberculosis (TB) is caused by *Mycobacterium tuberculosis. M. tuberculosis* is an extracellular agent and needs oxygen. It is attracted to the upper respiratory tract. It is also a facultative intracellular invader and is able to evade the immune system. The immune system of the host attempts to control the spread of the bacterium by walling it off with macrophages. This causes a positive skin reaction (cell-mediated immune response) but no infection. TB is particularly dangerous to immunocompromised individuals. Symptoms of TB may include weight loss, general debility, night sweats, and fever. A progressive cough with dyspnea and bloody sputum is common in pulmonary involvement. The disease is transmitted through airborne particles. These particles suspend in the air and are inhaled. The following steps can be taken to prevent the spread of the disease: prompt diagnosis; administration of antituberculosis drugs; airborne infection isolation, skin testing, and x-rays for exposed individuals; and preventive isoniazid therapy for those with latent infection or those newly converted to positive on TB testing.

Asthma

An acute *asthma* attack occurs as a result of a precipitating stimulus, such as a substance that triggers an allergic response. An inflammatory cascade results that causes edema of the mucous membranes (swollen airway), contraction of smooth muscles (bronchospasm), increased mucus production (cough and obstruction), and hyperinflation of the airways (decreased ventilation and shunting). Mast cells and T lymphocytes produce cytokines. The cytokines cause increased blood flow, vasoconstriction, and bronchoconstriction. This causes fluid to leak from the blood vessels. Epithelial cells and cilia are destroyed, exposing nerves and causing hypersensitivity. Bronchodilation is stimulated by sympathetic nervous system receptors in the bronchi. The three main symptoms of asthma are cough, wheezing, and dyspnea. In cough-variant asthma, a severe cough may be the only symptom at the onset of the condition.

There are a number of pharmacologic agents used in the treatment of asthma:
- Methylxanthines (aminophylline and theophylline) stimulate muscle contractions of the chest and stimulate respirations.
- Magnesium sulfate is used to relax smooth muscles and decrease inflammation. These drugs may be administered intravenously or by inhalation. If given intravenously, magnesium sulfate must be administered slowly to prevent the occurrence of hypotension or bradycardia. When inhaled, the drug potentiates the action of albuterol.
- Heliox (helium-oxygen) is given to decrease airway resistance in cases of airway obstruction. It works to decrease respiratory effort. Heliox improves oxygenation in patients requiring mechanical ventilation.
- Leukotriene inhibitors are used in the long-term management of asthma and inhibit inflammation and bronchospasm. *Cromolyn sodium* and nedocromil may be administered to prevent asthmatic response to exercise or allergens.

Agents Used in Pulmonary Pharmacology

There are a wide range of agents used in pulmonary pharmacology. The agents used depend on the type and degree of pulmonary disease.
- Opioid analgesics are given to provide pain relief and sedation for those on mechanical ventilation. These agents reduce sympathetic response. Such medications include fentanyl

(Sublimaze) or morphine sulfate (MS Contin).

- Neuromuscular blockers are used to induce paralysis in individuals who have not responded adequately to sedation, especially for the purposes of intubation and mechanical ventilation. Medications include pancuronium (Pavulon) and vecuronium (Norcuron). There is controversy surrounding the use of these drugs because induced paralysis has been linked to increased mortality rates, sensory hearing loss (pancuronium), atelectasis, and ventilation-perfusion mismatch.
- Human B-type natriuretic peptides are used to lower pulmonary capillary wedge pressure. Medications include nesiritide (Natrecor).
- Vasopressors/inotropes are used to raise cardiac output. Dopamine (Intropin) increases renal output and blood pressure. Dobutamine (Dobutrex) increases cardiac contractibility and blood pressure.
- Surfactants lower surface tension and prevent alveoli from collapsing. Beractant (Survanta) is made from bovine lung tissue, and calfactant (Infasurf) is made from calf lung tissue. These agents are administered by inhalation.
- Alkalinizers are used in the treatment of metabolic acidosis. These drugs reduce pulmonary vascular resistance by producing an alkaline pH. Medications include sodium bicarbonate and tromethamine (Tham). Administered by inhalation.
- nitrous oxide is used as a pulmonary vasodilator. This gas relaxes the vascular muscles and produces pulmonary vasodilation. The gas may reduce the need for extracorporeal membrane oxygenation (ECMO).
- Methylxanthines are used to stimulate contractions of the chest muscles and stimulate respiration. Medications

include aminophylline.(Aminophylline), caffeine citrate (Cafcit), and doxapram (Dopram).
- Diuretics are used to decrease pulmonary edema. Agents include loop diuretics, such as furosemide (Lasix) and metolazone (Mykrox).
- Nitrates are administered for the purpose of vasodilation. Vasodilation reduces preload and afterload, which reduces the heart muscle's oxygen requirement. Nitrates include nitroglycerin (Nitro-Bid) and nitroprusside sodium (Nitropress).
- Antibiotics are used to treat respiratory infections, including pneumonia. Antibiotics used depend on the pathogenic agent in question and may include macrolides such as azithromycin (Zithromax) and erythromycin (E-Mycin).
- Antimycobacterials are used to treat tuberculosis and other mycobacterial diseases. Antimycobacterial agents include isoniazid (Laniazid, Nydrazid), ethambutol (Myambutol), rifampin (Rifadin), streptomycin sulfate, and pyrazinamide.
- Antivirals are used to disrupt viral replication early in a viral infection. The effectiveness of this treatment decreases with time because the replication process is already under way. Antiviral medications include ribavirin (Virazole) and zanamivir (Relenza).

Laxative Products

There are different types of laxatives: Stool softeners (emollients, such as Colace and Phillips' Liqui-Gels) use wetting agents, such as docusate sodium, to increase liquid in the stool. The increased liquid softens the stool. Stool softeners should not be used in conjunction with mineral oil because of increased absorption of the oil through the intestines. Hyperosmotics, which are available by prescription, contain materials that are not digestible and keep stool moist by holding fluid in the stool. Hyperosmotics (such as Kristalose and MiraLAX) soften the stool but may result in increased abdominal distention and flatus. There are three types of hyperosmolar laxatives: 1) lactulose: . Lactulose hyperosmotics contain a form of sugar and work similarly to saline laxatives, but more slowly, and may be used for long-term treatment, 2) polymer: The polymers contain polyethylene glycol, which retains fluid in the stool and is used for short-term relief, and 3) saline: The salines work quickly and are used for short-term relief. Combination drugs use two or more types of laxatives and should be used only for short-term treatment.

Medical Treatments

Medical treatments for fecal incontinence include the following:

Medications
- Antidiarrheals: reduce diarrhea, increase rectal muscle tone, decrease stool fluid content, and protect the lining of the intestine from irritation.
- Cholinergic medications: reduce intestinal motility and secretions. Opium derivatives increase intestinal muscle tone and decrease motility.
- Laxatives: treat constipation.
- Stool softeners: increase the amount of fluid in the stool.
- Rectal stimulants: cause bowel contractions to increase, leading to increased stool evacuation.
- Hormones: are administered to postmenopausal women to improve incontinence.

Diet:
High-fiber products are recommended to absorb fluid and add bulk. Food allergies or intolerances (lactose intolerance, for example) are evaluated, and irritating foods are removed from the diet.

Bowel training:
Bowel training combines the use of medication, diet, and enemas to aid in evacuation of the bowels.

Biofeedback:
Biofeedback trains people to respond to rectal distention. It involves contraction of the pelvic floor and external sphincter muscle.

Procon incontinence device:
The Procon incontinent device is a catheter with a sensor; it is inserted into the rectum with an inflatable balloon to prevent leakage.

Bowel Obstruction and Infarction

Bowel obstruction can occur for the following reasons: an obstruction of the passage of intestinal contents because of constriction of the lumen, occlusion of the lumen, or lack of muscular contractions (paralytic ileus). Obstruction may be caused by congenital or acquired abnormality. Symptoms of bowel obstruction include abdominal pain and distention, abdominal rigidity, vomiting and dehydration, diminished or absent bowel sounds, severe constipation (obstipation), respiratory distress (resulting from pressure exerted by the diaphragm), shock (resulting from diminishing plasma volume and the movement of electrolytes from the bloodstream into the intestines), and sepsis (resulting from bacteria proliferation in the bowel and invasion of the bloodstream by bacteria).

Bowel infarction is ischemia of the intestines resulting from a severely restricted blood supply. It can be the result of a number of different conditions, such as strangulated bowel or occlusion of arteries of the mesentery. It may occur subsequent to untreated bowel obstruction. Patients present with acute abdomen and shock. The mortality rate is very high even with resection of the infarcted section of bowel.

Contributing Factors

Bowel dysfunction can be caused by factors that can be corrected and factors that require compensation. Bowel dysfunction includes diarrhea, constipation, and gas. Dietary factors that can contribute to bowel dysfunction include insufficient fiber and fluids and ingestion of certain foods. Some clinical conditions (such as hemorrhoids) may cause pain that delays defecation. Surgical treatment of hemorrhoids, fistulas, or the rectum may cause injury to the sphincters. Chronic diseases (such as irritable bowel syndrome and multiple sclerosis) may be associated with bowel dysfunction. Dementia may be associated with the inability to manage toileting. Delay of defecation is the most common cause of constipation, impaction, and fecal incontinence. Delay of defecation may result from functional disability or dementia. Medications frequently cause constipation. Some medications (antacids and antibiotics, for example) can cause diarrhea. Laxative abuse results in the development of laxative tolerance. Physical inactivity reduces bowel motility and increases constipation.

Diarrhea

Diarrhea is a condition in which an individual passes liquid or semi-liquid stool more frequently than is normal. Diarrhea is often accompanied by abdominal cramping, distention, and sense of urgency to defecate. Individuals with severe diarrhea may need to defecate hourly. Diarrhea is characterized according to color, odor, consistency, and frequency of defecation. Diarrhea may be acute or chronic. *Acute diarrhea* usually has a sudden onset and may be caused by chemotherapy, irritating foods, gastrointestinal organisms, and stress. Diarrhea may be watery or bloody. It may be accompanied by flatus. Acute diarrhea usually

resolves without treatment within a few days or responds to anti-diarrheals. *Chronic diarrhea* persists more than three days and is usually the result of a long-term disease process (such as Crohn's disease) or trauma (such as radiation therapy). Certain foods may irritate the gastrointestinal tract and cause chronic diarrhea. Chronic diarrhea may also result from laxative overuse, in which there may be a cycle of constipation followed by diarrhea.

Constipation is a condition in which bowel movements are abnormally infrequent for an individual or in which hard, small stools are evacuated from the bowels fewer than three times per week. Food travels from the small intestine to the colon in semi-liquid form. Fluid is absorbed in the colon, which is responsible for the consistency of the stool. If too much fluid is absorbed, the stool can become too dry. An individual with constipation may have abdominal distention and cramps and need to strain for defecation.

Fecal impaction occurs when hard stool in the rectum becomes a large, dense, immovable mass that cannot be expelled even with straining. Fecal impaction usually occurs as a result of chronic constipation. A person with fecal impaction may experience abdominal cramps and distention and intense rectal pressure and pain. The individual may feel a sense of urgency to defecate. Symptoms may include nausea and vomiting. In a case of fecal impaction, hemorrhoids will often become engorged. Fecal incontinence, with liquid stool leaking out around the impaction, may occur.

Risk Factors

Common risk factors for fecal incontinence include the following:
- Age: Fecal incontinence is most common among elderly people with health problems, such as urinary incontinence.

- Sex: Women are more likely than men to experience fecal incontinence because women often suffer damage to the sphincter during childbirth. For example, scar tissue that forms after episiotomy may cause fecal incontinence. In addition, muscles weaken after multiple childbirths.
- Neurological damage: Congenital or acquired neurological defects are highly associated with fecal incontinence. In addition, progressive neuropathy (such as diabetes mellitus or multiple sclerosis) may result in the inability to control defecation.
- Dementia/Alzheimer's disease: Both fecal and urinary incontinence occur in late-stage Alzheimer's disease.
- Physical disability: Physical disability, either congenital or acquired, may lead to fecal incontinence. Accessing a toilet may be difficult for individuals with a disability. Some individuals may be unable to express the need to defecate. Others may not be able to physically manage toileting without assistance.

Malnutrition Risks

There are a number of risk factors for malnutrition. Hyper-metabolism can result from various diseases (acquired immunodeficiency syndrome [AIDS], for example) and other conditions (such as stress). It can also result from trauma. Weight loss is a risk factor for malnutrition, especially a sudden weight loss or the loss of 10 percent of normal weight over a three-month period. Low body weight (less than 90 percent of the ideal body weight for age) is a risk factor for malnutrition. Low body mass index (BMI) (less than 18.5) is associated with malnutrition. Immunosuppressive drugs can interfere with the absorption of nutrients. Malabsorption of nutrients may be caused by diseases such as chronic kidney or liver failure. Changes in appetite may decrease intake of nutrients. Food intolerances may

result from lack of enzymes necessary to digest certain foods. Dietary restrictions, such as the need to limit protein intake with kidney failure, can result in malnutrition. Functional limitations may impair the ability to take in nutrients. The lack of teeth or functioning dentures may limit food intake. Alterations in taste and smell may render food unpalatable.

Nutritional Assessment

Physical assessment is an important part of nutritional assessment. Physical impairment may affect nutritional status. Hair may be dry, brittle, or thinning. Skin may exhibit poor turgor or ecchymosis. Tears, pressure areas, ulcerations, abrasions, or other compromises may be present. The mouth may display dry mucous membranes. The lips may have cheilosis and cracking at the corners. Lips may be scaly (riboflavin deficiency). Gums may be swollen or bleeding. The teeth may be loose or need care. Dentures may fit poorly. The tongue may be inflamed, dry, cracked, or have sores. Nails may become brittle. A spoon-shaped or pale nail bed indicates low iron. Hands may be crippled or arthritic, making eating difficult. Vision may be compromised, interfering with the ability to prepare food or to eat. Mental status may be impaired enough that the affected individual can't understand diet instructions or prepare or eat meals. Motor skills may decrease, including hand/mouth coordination. The ability to hold utensils may be impaired.

Dehydration

Older adults do not conserve water efficiently, have a less pronounced sense of thirst, and may have impaired sodium balance. Lean body mass in an older adult decreases from 65 percent to 40 percent; fat increases and total body water decreases. Dehydration results when total body water decreases but total body sodium does not decrease. This can result from inadequate fluid intake, excess water loss, disease, nasogastric suctioning, drugs, diarrhea, vomiting, and fever. Diagnostic criteria include increased hematocrit, blood urea nitrogen (BUN)/creatinine ratio, and sodium (greater than 20 mEq/L). Treatment includes estimating fluid loss and replacing 50 percent of the loss within the first 12 hours. Dehydration can be mild, moderate, or severe:

- Mild dehydration: involves a five percent loss of total body water. Symptoms include dizziness, lethargy, altered mentation, decreased skin turgor, dry mucous membranes, dysrhythmia, and orthostatic hypotension. Treatment includes increasing oral fluids or the administration of intravenous fluids.
- Moderate dehydration: involves a 10 percent loss of total body water. Symptoms include confusion, resting hypotension, tachycardia, and oliguria/anuria.
- Severe dehydration: involves a greater than 15 percent loss of total body water. Marked hypotension and anuria occur at this stage.

Dental Conditions in the Elderly

Approximately 28 percent of individuals younger than age 75 are edentulous, while 43 percent of individuals older than age 75 are edentulous. Some edentulous individuals wear dentures, but others eventually stop wearing dentures due to poor fit or because the dentures have caused oral lesions (30%). If patients have had the same dentures for a number of years, the dentures may need to be refitted or replaced. Approximately one-third of older adults have untreated caries. Frequently, these are root caries, which occur because of the recession of gum tissue. Gum-tissue recession occurs in about 86 percent of those older than age 65. Gum-tissue recession leaves the roots exposed and increases the risk of developing periodontal disease. Periodontal disease affects about 85 percent of older adults with 25 percent exhibiting loss

of supporting structures. Periodontal disease is characterized by pockets of swollen, bleeding, erythematous gingiva around the teeth. Effective oral hygiene, including brushing and flossing, use of mouthwashes, and cleaning, is important in combating periodontal disease. Surgical treatment may be required.

Dysphagia

Dysphagia is exhibited as difficulty swallowing solids and thin liquids. It occurs in approximately 10 percent of non-institutionalized older adults. Symptoms of the disorder include tightness or pain in the chest, regurgitation, choking, esophageal reflux, and aspiration pneumonia. Dysphagia may result in weight loss and dehydration. Diagnosis of the disorder is based on symptoms, barium swallow, and endoscopy. The patient is instructed to eat sitting upright, avoid eating before lying down, chew foods slowly, sip water after swallowing, thicken thin liquids, and limit bite size. The variety of underlying causes must be treated:

- Stroke: Approximately 30 percent of stroke patients have dysphagia.
- Neuromuscular diseases: Individuals with Parkinson's disease, myasthenia gravis, multiple sclerosis, and amyotrophic lateral sclerosis (ALS) may have dysphagia.
- Drugs: Phenothiazines may cause dysphagia.
- Dementia: Individuals with dementia may not chew food sufficiently or may neglect to swallow.
- Achalasia: If the esophagus does not contract effectively and the sphincter does not relax, then dysphagia can result.
- Esophageal stricture, diverticulum, or web (from iron deficiency) may lead to dysphagia.
- Esophageal cancer causes dysphagia.

Ulcers

Peptic Ulcers

A gastrointestinal (GI) hemorrhage (peptic ulcers)may occur in either the upper or lower GI tract. The main cause of GI hemorrhage (50 to 70% of cases) is peptic ulcer disease (gastric and duodenal ulcers). Peptic ulcer disease causes the gastromucosal lining to break down, which compromises the glycoprotein mucous barrier and the gastroduodenal epithelial cells that provide protection from gastric secretions. The gastric secretions erode the mucosal and submucosal layers, damaging blood vessels and causing hemorrhage. The primary causes are nonsteroidal anti-inflammatory drugs (NSAIDs) and infection by the Helicobacter pylori bacterium. Symptoms include abdominal pain and distention, bloody or tarry stools, hypotension, and tachycardia. Treatment includes fluid replacement; antibiotic therapy for H. pylori infection; endoscopic thermal therapy to cauterize; injection therapy (hypertonic saline, epinephrine, and ethanol) to cause vasoconstriction; and arteriography with intra-arterial infusion of vasopressin and/or embolizing agents (such as stainless steel coils, platinum microcoils, or Gelfoam pledgets). A vagotomy and pyloroplasty are performed if bleeding persists.

Stress Ulcers

Stress-related erosive syndrome (SRES—stress ulcers) occurs most often in individuals with critical illnesses (individuals with severe or multiorgan trauma, mechanical ventilation, sepsis, severe burns, and head injury with increased intracranial pressure). Stress causes changes in the gastric mucosal lining and a decrease in perfusion of the mucosa. These changes cause ischemia. Hemorrhage occurs in more than 30 percent of individuals with SRES, with a mortality rate of 30 to 80 percent. This makes prompt identification and treatment critical. The lesions associated with SRES tend to be diffuse and are more difficult to treat than peptic ulcers. Symptoms include coffee-grounds emesis, hematemesis, and abdominal discomfort. There are prophylactic treatments for those at risk of the disorder. Sucralfate (Carafate) protects mucosa against pepsin. Famotidine (Pepcid), nizatidine (Axid), ranitidine (Zantac), and cimetidine (Tagamet) reduce gastric secretions. Treatment for active bleeding includes intra-arterial infusion of vasopressin and intra-arterial embolization. Oversewing of ulcers or total gastrectomy is performed if bleeding persists.

Hiatal Hernias

The esophagus exits the pleural cavity and enters the abdominal cavity through an opening in the diaphragm. The diaphragm should surround the esophagus tightly to prevent the stomach from entering the pleural cavity. A hiatal hernia results when a defect in the diaphragm causes it to loosen and permits a portion of the stomach to swell into the chest cavity. Hiatal hernias occur more often in women than in men. There are two main types of hiatal hernia: sliding and paraesophageal (rolling). Some individuals may have a combined form. A *sliding hiatal hernia* occurs when the gastroesophageal junction and the proximal stomach slide in and out of the chest cavity. This is the most common form (about 90%) of hiatal hernia. A sliding hiatal hernia occurs because of a laxity in the gastroesophageal junction, and the condition often involves reflux, regurgitation, and heartburn. A *paraesophageal hiatal hernia* is one in which all or part of the stomach swells up into the chest cavity while the gastroesophageal junction remains in place. This does not cause symptoms of reflux.

Gastroesophageal Reflux Disease

Gastroesophageal reflux disease (GERD) is the regurgitation of the stomach contents into the esophagus. It usually results from decreased tone in the gastroesophageal valve and hiatal hernia. The stomach contents damage the mucosal lining of the esophagus. A number of conditions may develop from GERD. These include chronic esophagitis, strictures, Barrett's esophagus (abnormal changes in the cells of the distal esophagus), and esophageal cancer. GERD symptoms include epigastric pain, heartburn, dysphagia, chronic cough (particularly at night), hoarseness, earache, and sinusitis. There are a number of treatments. Patients are advised to avoid eating large meals and snacking after dinner. Eating at least three hours before bedtime is recommended.

Certain foods, such as coffee, alcohol, fatty foods, spicy foods, and cruciferous vegetables, should be avoided. The patient is advised to sleep on the left side with the head of the bed elevated. The condition is also treated with medications, including histamine-2 receptor blockers (famotidine and ranitidine), proton pump inhibitors, alginic acid (Gaviscon), and antacids (without aluminum). Surgical repair, called fundoplication, may be necessary.

Small Intestine Cancers

The small intestine does not develop cancerous lesions as frequently as other parts of the gastrointestinal tract. The four main types of primary small intestine cancer are named according to the type of cells from which they develop:

- Adenocarcinomas are the most commonly occurring type of primary small intestine cancer. It originates in the lining of intestine and usually occurs in the duodenum.
- Carcinoids originate in hormone-producing cells in the small bowel. It occurs most frequently in the ileum and sometimes in the appendix.
- Lymphomas originate in the lymph tissue. They are generally of the non-Hodgkin's type and occur most frequently in the jejunum or ileum.
- Sarcomas originate in the supportive tissues, such as fat and muscle.

- Leiomyosarcomas generally develop in the muscle wall of the ileum.
- Gastrointestinal stromal tumors may originate in any section of the small intestine.

Colorectal Cancers

Adenocarcinomas, which account for 90 to 95 percent of colorectal cancers, originate in epithelial tissue in adenomatous polyps. There are two subtypes. Signet ring is a very aggressive form of adenocarcinoma. It is hard to treat but accounts for only 0.1 percent of adenocarcinomas. Mucinous is also an aggressive form of adenocarcinoma. This form is composed of about 60 percent mucus, which allows the cells to spread faster and makes the cancer difficult to treat. Mucinous adenocarcinoma accounts for 10 to 15 percent of adenocarcinomas. Sarcomas (leiomyosarcomas) develop in smooth muscle. Sarcomas account for less than two percent of colorectal cancers; however, over 50 percent of sarcomas metastasize. Carcinoids are slow-growing tumors that rarely spread and are most frequently found in the rectum. Carcinoids account for less than one percent of colorectal cancers. Lymphoma is a rare type of colorectal cancer. Lymphomas are primary tumors that usually occur in the rectum, while secondary metastatic tumors usually occur in the colon. This is a rare type of cancer. Melanomas are tumors that have usually metastasized from other parts of body. They account for less than two percent of colorectal cancers.

Ascending Colon Cancer

Stool enters the cecum and ascending colon in liquid form; therefore, cancers arising in these areas may grow to a large size before they cause obstruction and obvious symptoms. Lesions frequently ulcerate the intestine and cause chronic bleeding that may not change the character or the appearance of the stool. Liquid stool is able to pass through a very narrow opening. Twenty-two percent of colorectal tumors originate in the ascending colon. Symptoms include the following:

- Fatigue
- Generalized weakness
- Pallor
- Dull abdominal pain
- Loss of appetite
- Weight loss
- Occult blood or melena (tarry stools)
- Hypochromic microcytic anemia
- Chronic iron deficiency anemia
- Palpitations (related to anemia)
- Congestive heart failure (related to anemia)
- Palpable abdominal mass (may be evident with large tumors)
- Chronic diarrhea (may result with some large right-sided lesions)
- Bowel obstruction (in the late stages).

Transverse, Descending, Sigmoid, and Rectal Cancers

Fluid in the intestines is absorbed in the ascending colon, so stool in the transverse and descending colon is more solid. Lesions originating in the transverse and descending colon are usually annular constrictive lesions. These encircle the intestine and cause to obstruction. Tumors of the sigmoid colon and rectum may exert pressure on adjacent structures (such as the vagina, prostate, and bladder).

Characteristics of transverse and descending colon cancers include changes in bowel habits; abdominal cramping, especially in the left-lower quadrant; pencil-thin stools from narrowing of the lumen; constipation; abdominal distention; intestinal obstruction; perforation of the bowel; and peritonitis.

Characteristics of sigmoid colon and rectal cancers include tenesmus (painful, ineffective straining to pass stool); pain in rectal or perianal area; feeling of fullness and incomplete evacuation of stool; alternating constipation and diarrhea; frank blood in stool; blood clots; pencil-thin stools from narrowing of the lumen; abdominal pain and cramping; urinary symptoms; and vaginal fistulae.

Types of Cirrhosis

Cirrhosis of the liver is a condition in which the liver is scarred. The two types of cirrhosis are compensated and decompensated. The term compensated means that the liver is still capable of coping with the damage. In this case, there is no sign of liver failure.

Compensated cirrhosis is usually indicated by nonspecific symptoms, such as intermittent fever, epistaxis, edema, indigestion, abdominal pain, and palmar erythema. Hepatomegaly and splenomegaly may also be present. Many people with compensated cirrhosis are stable for years before the liver starts to fail. Liver failure does not occur suddenly, but slowly. Signs that the liver is starting to fail are evident for some time before failure occurs.

Decompensated cirrhosis occurs when the liver is no longer capable of synthesizing proteins, clotting factors, and other necessary substances. It is indicated by the development of one or more of the following symptoms: jaundice (yellow discoloration of the skin and eyes), variceal hemorrhage, fluid in the peritoneal cavity (ascites), and encephalopathy.

Liver Failure and Portal Hypertension

The right and left hepatic arteries supply the liver with oxygenated blood. The liver also receives nutrient-rich blood from the intestinal tract via the portal vein. Blood from the portal vein is filtered in the liver. Pathogens and nutrients from the blood are absorbed and metabolized in the liver by the hepatocytes. The liver stores nutrients and excretes unwanted substances into the hepatic veins and inferior vena cava. In liver failure, portal hypertension impairs this process.

In portal hypertension, the portal vein becomes blocked, and blood flow is reduced. This increases blood pressure in the portal venous system, which is already compressed by cirrhotic changes. Because the liver cannot adequately filter the blood, increased pressure creates collateral blood vessels that bypass the obstruction. Unfiltered blood returns to the systemic circulation via the collateral vessels. Varices form in the esophagus and other areas as a result of the collateral vessels. Increased aldosterone causes sodium and fluid to be retained. Plasma albumin decreases, causing fluid to leak from the vascular system. Ascites results from this process.

Hepatorenal syndrome and hepatic encephalopathy are part of the syndrome of hepatic failure.
- Hepatorenal syndrome involves a marked decrease in renal blood flow resulting in azotemia (abnormal levels of nitrogenous substances). Sodium level falls and potassium level increases. The syndrome involves abnormalities in blood chemistry and clotting time. Hepatorenal syndrome is related to hepatic encephalopathy.
- Hepatic encephalopathy occurs when ammonia crosses the blood-brain barrier and is absorbed by brain tissue. Under normal circumstances, protein is digested in the intestines and the ammonia that is produced as a waste product is filtered by the liver and broken down to form urea. Restricted blood flow from the portal system causes the level of ammonia in the blood to increase. Ammonia causes mental confusion, stupor, and finally, coma. Marked changes are observable on an electroencephalogram (EEG).

Prostrate Gland

Prostatitis is an acute infection of the prostate gland. It is caused by bacteria such as *Escherichia coli, Pseudomonas*, or *Staphylococcus*. Symptoms include fever and chills lower back pain, frequent urination, dysuria, painful ejaculation, and perineal discomfort.

Diagnosis is based on physical assessment showing perineal tenderness and spasm of the rectal sphincter. Treatment includes 500 mg of ciprofloxacin taken orally twice a day for one month (treatment of choice) and trimethoprim/sulfamethoxazole double-strength (TMP/SMX DS) twice daily for one month. A urethral culture is taken to check for sexually transmitted diseases (STDs).

Benign prostatic hypertrophy/hyperplasia usually develops in men after the age of 40. The prostate enlarges gradually, but the surrounding tissue limits outward growth, so the gland compresses the urethra. The bladder wall also exhibits changes. It becomes thicker and irritated and begins to spasm, causing frequent urination. With time, the bladder muscle weakens and the bladder does not empty completely on urination. Symptoms include urgency, dribbling, frequent urination, nocturia, incontinence, urine retention, and bladder distention. Diagnostic methods include intravenous pyelogram (IVP), cystogram, and prostate-specific antigen (PSA). Treatment methods include catheterization for urine retention and surgical excision.

Bladder Cancer

Bladder cancer originates in the lining of the urinary organs and then invades the deeper layers. The bladder wall and lining of the urinary tract are composed of several layers, listed here from the inner to the outer layer: the urothelium (mucosa), urothelial (transitional) cells lining the inside layer of the urinary tract; the lamina propria (submucosa), a thin layer of connective tissue; the muscularis propria, a thicker layer of muscle; the serosa, fatty connective tissue covering the superior surfaces; and the adventitia, covering areas with no serosa.

There are several symptoms of bladder cancer. Gross hematuria is the presence of blood in the urine. Bright red blood may be evident. The urine may be brown or rust colored. The blood in the urine may appear intermittently. The patient may exhibit microscopic hematuria; in this case, the blood is visible only under a microscope. The patient may experience dysuria. Bladder cancer may cause burning or pain on urination and a feeling that the bladder does not empty completely. Urination may be frequent.

Sexual Dysfunction

Sexual activity lessens with age. However, approximately 50 percent of individuals older than age 60 engage in sexual activity. Typically, sexual desire decreases with age. Women have more difficulty reaching orgasm as they age. Vaginal lubrication decreases, and vaginal atrophy may be present. Men require more stimulation to achieve an erection, which may not be as firm. The amount of ejaculate may be decreased. *Dyspareunia* (painful intercourse) may be treated with vaginal estrogen preparations in the form of creams and tablets. Water-based products may be used to provide lubrication. *Erectile dysfunction* may result from vascular disease, diabetes, smoking, urinary tract infections (UTIs), alcohol use, obesity, and lack of testosterone. Various medications may also cause erectile dysfunction. Treatment may include oral medications (such as Viagra, Cialis), intracorporeal injections (injections into the corpus cavernosa), or intraurethral medications (pellets inserted into the urethra with an applicator). Mechanical devices to treat erectile dysfunction include external vacuum tumescence devices (an elastic ring at the base of the penis inhibits venous drainage to maintain erection) and the penile prosthesis (a surgical procedure used if other means fail).

Urinary Tract Infections

Urinary infections develop in the urinary tract (kidneys, ureters, bladder, and urethra). These are common and often recurring low-grade infections. The prompt treatment of urinary infections is very important. Some symptoms of urinary tract infection appear as changes in the character of the urine. The urine may become cloudy from mucus or purulent material. Blood may be evident in the urine. The urine may take on a dark yellow, orange, or brown color as it becomes more concentrated. The urine may have a very strong or foul odor. Urinary output may decrease markedly. A urinary tract infection may cause pain in the lower back or flank, resulting from inflammation of the kidneys. Systemic symptoms include fever, chills, headache, and general malaise. Some people suffer lack of appetite, nausea, and vomiting. Fever usually indicates that the infection has affected the kidneys. The treatment for urinary tract infection includes increased fluid intake and antibiotics.

Urinary Incontinence

There are many potential causes of urinary incontinence:
- Pregnancy/childbirth: Childbirth weakens the muscles of the pelvic floor and urethral sphincter. Nerve damage and bladder prolapse are also possible complications of pregnancy that can contribute to incontinence.
- Postmenopausal changes: Menopause involves a loss of estrogen. This can cause bladder and urethral tissues to weaken.
- Hysterectomy: This surgery can damage the muscles and nerves in the urinary tract because of the proximity of the urinary tract and the uterus.

- Interstitial cystitis: This is an inflammation that sometimes causes incontinence.
- Prostate enlargement: The enlarging prostate constricts the urethra and leads to urgency or overflow incontinence.
- Prostate cancer: Incontinence may be caused directly by the cancer or may occur in response to radiation or the surgical removal of the prostate.
- Bladder cancer: Dysuria and incontinence are common symptoms.
- Neurological deficits: Neurological deficits present at birth or caused by injury or disease can result in the inability to control urination.
- Urinary tract obstruction: An obstruction anywhere in the urinary tract can cause overflow incontinence.

Four Types of Urinary Incontinence

The different types of urinary incontinence are as follows: urge, stress, overflow, functional, reflex, mixed, and induced. An individual may have more than one type of incontinence.

- An individual with urge incontinence feels a pressing need to urinate as soon as the bladder feels full. As a result, the individual may urinate on the way to the toilet or in bed during the night. Diuretics may worsen urge incontinence.
- Stress incontinence involves a sudden increase in bladder pressure resulting from such actions as coughing, laughing, or bending. Stress incontinence causes small amount of urine to leak from the bladder. It is common in people who are obese.
- Overflow incontinence usually occurs when the bladder is overfull. Small amounts of urine dribble from the urinary tract. However, the leakage can be almost constant.
- Functional incontinence results from physical or mental impairment or environmental barriers to urination, such as the lack of an accessible bathroom.
- Reflex urination involves the loss of urine without the individual's awareness. It occurs as a result of a fistula or bladder leak.

Medical Treatments

The following are medical treatments for urinary incontinence:

Medications:
- Antispasmodics (Detrol, Ditropan, and Levsin): Antispasmodics are administered in the treatment of overactive bladders. These agents may cause thirst. Longer-acting preparations of these drugs have fewer side effects and may be more appropriate for some patients.
- Antidepressants (Tofranil): Antidepressants are administered to relax the bladder and to contract the muscles at the bladder neck. Hormone replacement therapy (HRT): HRT is used in the form of a vaginal cream, ring, or patch. Its purpose is to protect bladder and urethral mucosa. Oral estrogen may not be as effective as a topical preparation for the treatment of incontinence.
- Antibiotics: Infection may cause or worsen incontinence. Antibiotics are administered to treat these infections.

Medical devices:
- Catheters: Intermittent catheterization may be used to empty the bladder.
- Penile clamps: These devices exert pressure around the penis and clamp the urethra.
- Pessary: A pessary is a stiff ring inserted vaginally to treat bladder prolapse.
- Urethral inserts: Urethral inserts are inserted temporarily into the urethra before activities that may trigger incontinence.

Pyelonephritis

Pyelonephritis is a bacterial infection of the parenchyma of the kidney. The infection has the potential to permanently damage the kidneys. Pyelonephritis can lead to abscess formation, sepsis, and kidney failure. Pyelonephritis is especially dangerous to individuals who have compromised immune systems, are pregnant, or have diabetes. Most infections are caused by *Escherichia coli*. Symptoms vary widely but can include dysuria, frequent urination, hematuria, flank and/or low-back pain, fever and chills, costovertebral angle tenderness, and changes in mental status (geriatric). Patients may need to be hospitalized and require careful follow-up. Diagnosis is based on urinalysis and blood and urine cultures. Treatments include analgesia, antipyretics, intravenous fluids, and antibiotics. Antibiotics used to treat pyelonephritis include ceftriaxone and fluoroquinolone.

Renal Failure

Renal failure is the inability of the kidneys to filter waste products, excrete waste products, concentrate urine, and maintain electrolyte balance. Renal failure may occur because of hypoxia, kidney disease, or obstruction of the urinary tract. It leads to azotemia (accumulation of nitrogenous waste in the blood) followed by uremia (toxic symptoms caused by accumulation of nitrogenous wastes). The kidneys cannot perform necessary functions after 50 percent of functional renal capacity is lost. Loss of renal function leads to progressive deterioration and eventually end-stage renal disease. Initial symptoms are often nonspecific and include loss of appetite, loss of energy, weight loss, muscle cramping, fatigue, bruising of the skin, dry or itching skin, increase in blood urea nitrogen (BUN) and serum creatinine, fluid retention (leading to edema), hyperkalemia, metabolic acidosis, calcium and phosphorus depletion (leading to altered bone structure and metabolism), and uremic syndrome.

Treatment for renal failure includes dialysis and transplantation. The patient receives supportive care and symptomatic therapy.

Vulvovaginitis

Vulvovaginitis is a condition in which the vulva and vaginal tissues are inflamed. There are a number of different causes: bacterial (*Gardnerella vaginalis*), fungal (usually *Candida albicans*), or parasitic (*Trichomonas vaginalis*). Vulvovaginitis can be caused by an allergy to soaps or other irritants (allergic-contact vaginitis). In addition, atrophic vaginitis occurs in women who are postmenopausal. Symptoms of the condition include vaginal odor, swelling, discharge, bleeding, pain, and itching. Diagnosis is based on physical examination, culture (discharge), and pH testing. Treatment depends on the cause of the condition. Bacterial infections are treated with all of the following medications simultaneously: metronidazole orally, metronidazole gel intravaginally, and clindamycin cream. Fungal infections are treated with Diflucan or vaginal creams, tablets, or suppositories (such as Femstat or Vagistat). Parasitic (*Trichomonas*) infections are treated with metronidazole orally.

Anemia

Anemia is an abnormally low level of normal red blood cells or hemoglobin. Anemia is often caused by hemorrhage, hemolysis, hematopoiesis, or iron deficiency (in menstruating women). Anemia causes a decrease in oxygen transportation and a decrease in perfusion. This causes the heart to increase cardiac output. The blood becomes less viscous, and peripheral resistance decreases. More blood is pumped to the heart. The turbulence that results from the increased blood flow can cause a heart murmur and, perhaps, heart failure. Symptoms of anemia include general malaise and weakness, loss of appetite, pallor, shortness of breath on exertion, headache, dizziness, depression, decreased attention span, slowed cognitive processes, shock symptoms (with severe blood loss), tachycardia, hypotension, and poor peripheral circulation. Treatment includes identification of the cause, blood or blood components as indicated, oxygen, and intravenous fluids. A splenectomy may be performed for hemolytic anemias.

Leukemia

Effects of Leukemia on Blood and Bone Marrow

In about 80 percent of cases, leukemia in older adults is *acute myelogenous leukemia* (AML). This condition may be associated with a history of radiation or chemotherapy. However, most cases are idiopathic. The cancer cells compete with normal cells for nutrition. Older adults often exhibit the following signs and symptoms: fever, malaise, pallor, weakness, and confusion. In every type of leukemia, all cells are affected because the cancer cells in the bone marrow depress the formation of all elements. This has the following results: a decrease in production of erythrocytes (red blood cells [RBCs]), resulting in anemia; a decrease in neutrophils, resulting in increased risk of infection; a decrease in platelets, with subsequent decrease in clotting factors and increased bleeding (nosebleeds are common); and an increased risk of physiological fractures because of a weakening of the periosteum.

Effects of Leukemia on Organs, the Central Nervous System and Metabolism

There are numerous effects of leukemia. The liver, spleen, and lymph glands are infiltrated, resulting in enlargement and fibrosis. Infiltration of the central nervous system (CNS) results in increased intracranial pressure, ventricular dilation, and meningeal irritation. These reactions cause headaches, vomiting, papilledema, nuchal rigidity, and coma progressing to death. Hypermetabolism is exhibited. This deprives cells of nutrients and results in anorexia, weight loss, muscle

atrophy, and fatigue. Treatment (chemotherapy) is more difficult in older adults who may not tolerate the pancytopenia. The goal of treatment in this age group is remission. Bone marrow transplantation is usually performed only in individuals younger than age 65. Infections requiring antibiotic therapy are common with leucopenia. Such infections compromise already-weakened patients. Regardless of the aggressiveness of treatment, older adults often relapse within a year and die one to two years following diagnosis. Therefore, treatment options depend on age, general condition, and potential outcome. Palliative care is often indicated.

Osteoporosis

Osteoporosis is a condition involving low bone mass and structural deterioration. More bone is lost than gained. The condition leads to thin, porous bones that break easily. Osteoporosis occurs most commonly in postmenopausal women, although men older than age 65 experience bone loss at the same rate as women. Primary osteoporosis occurs as part of normal aging. Bone mass density (BMD) can be tested to determine the extent of osteoporosis. The risk factors for osteoporosis can be arranged to spell the word FRACTURED and are as follows:

- **f**ractures,
- **r**ace,
- **a**ge and gender,
- **c**hronic disease/medication,
- **t**hin bones and low weight,
- **u**nderactive/inadequate exercise,
- **r**educed estrogen,
- **e**xcessive alcohol intake and smoking, and
  diet.

Cancer survivors and individuals with chronic disease are at increased risk for osteoporosis. Treatments include the following medications: bisphosphonates, hormones (not recommended), selective estrogen receptor modulator, calcitonin, and recombinant human parathyroid hormone. A diet high in calcium and vitamin D may be recommended. Balance training, strength training, and regular weight-bearing exercise will often improve symptoms of osteoporosis.

Gait and Mobility Issues

Approximately 20 percent of noninstitutionalized adults and 54 percent of institutionalized adults older than age 85 have gait and mobility issues that limit their independence and predispose them to falls. Risk factors include arthritis, peripheral neuropathy, hypothyroidism, Parkinson's disease, orthostatic hypotension, deformities, stroke and heart attack, medication effects, and orthopedic problems. Weakness, loss of muscle mass and tone, and confusion may contribute to gait disorders. An older patient should be observed for gait abnormalities, including unsteadiness, uneven weight distribution, and abnormal positioning of limbs. A slow gait, covering five meters in less than 0.6 m/second, is predictive of functional limitations. In the Timed Up and Go (TUG) test, the patient stands from a sitting position in a chair with armrests, walks three meters and turns, walks back to the chair, and sits down again. Those requiring 14 seconds or more are at risk for falls. The Performance Oriented Mobility Assessment (POMA) tests mobility and gait under different conditions. Treatment for mobility issues includes identifying and treating the underlying cause, gait and strength training, environmental modifications, assistive devices, and orthotics.

Osteoarthritis and Rheumatoid Arthritis

Osteoarthritis often occurs following injury, but it may be idiopathic. The disease is progressive, with symptoms occurring after age 60. Osteoarthritis involves deterioration of the cartilage. Signs and symptoms of the disease include increasing pain with use and/or weight bearing and stiffness. The involvement is local and unilateral. Treatment includes nonsteroidal anti-inflammatory drugs (NSAIDs), heat, weight reduction, joint rest, orthotic devices, postural exercises, osteotomy, and arthroplasty (with joint replacement).

Rheumatoid arthritis is a systemic autoimmune inflammatory disorder. Its cause is unknown. It has an acute onset, and is first evident in the hands, wrists, and feet. The disease develops between the ages of 25 to 50 years. Rheumatoid arthritis causes joint inflammation and deformity. Signs and symptoms include pain, stiffness, swelling, erythema, nodules, generalized weakness, fatigue, weight loss, and fever. The involvement is systemic, bilateral, and symmetric. Treatment includes light exercise to prevent contractures. Medications used to treat the disease include salicylates (ASA), NSAIDs, cyclo-oxygenase-2 (COX-2) inhibitors (Celebrex), disease-modifying antirheumatic drugs (gold-containing compounds, methotrexate, azathioprine, and adalimumab), immunomodulators (abatacept), interleukin 1 receptor inhibitors (anakinra), and glucocorticoids (prednisone) and topical analgesics.

Hip Fracture

Falls occur in 30 percent of those older than age 65, and 50 percent of those older than age 80. About five percent of these falls result in fractures. Hip fractures pose the greatest risk to the older adult. Osteoporosis increases risk of fracture. Bone deterioration may cause pain in the hip, and the patient may have difficulty bearing weight prior to a fall. The most common fracture sites are the femoral neck and the intertrochanteric region. Patients may have comorbidities and may present with dehydration and blood loss. The mortality rate is 10 percent during initial treatment and 25 percent or more over the next year. Various types of repair are performed, including cannulated screw fixation, internal fixation, total hip replacement, extramedullary implant (sliding screw and plate), intramedullary implant

(Gamma nail), or hip compression screw and side plate. Yearly infusion of Reclast started within three months of a fracture has been shown to reduce the incidence of new fractures and to increase survival rate.

Musculoskeletal Deformities

Musculoskeletal deformities occur frequently in older adults and may interfere with mobility and independence or cause serious health problems. Bones become more porous, muscle mass reduces, and ligaments and tendons lose strength and elasticity. Foot deformities (such as bunions, hammertoes, corns, calluses, and bone spurs) may cause pain and inflammation and limit mobility. Hand deformities (such as those caused by arthritis or carpal tunnel syndrome) may increase dependence. Overuse syndromes and decreased sensation of touch are common. The hands may feel cold due to vascular insufficiency. Spinal deformities include kyphosis, lordosis, and scoliosis. *Kyphosis* is a convex angulation of the thoracic spine. It may occur as a consequence of arthritis or compression fractures. Kyphosis may cause compression of thoracic and abdominal structures and lead to decreased ventilation and perfusion. *Lordosis* is a frequently painful concave angulation of the lumbar spine. It is often associated with obesity, flexion hip contracture, and slipped femoral capital epiphysis. *Scoliosis* is a lateral and rotational curvature of the spine. It can cause alterations in the structure of the pelvis and chest.

Diabetes

Type 1 Diabetes
The most commonly occurring metabolic disorder is diabetes mellitus. Type 1 diabetes is an autoimmune disease. Insufficient insulin production occurs as a result of the destruction of pancreatic beta cells. This results in a lack of insulin. The lack of insulin first leads to an increase in fasting blood glucose and then to an increase in urine glucose. Individuals with the disorder exhibit pronounced polyuria and polydipsia. The disease has a fast onset. Individuals with the disorder may be overweight or have experienced a recent weight loss. Ketoacidosis may be present. Insulin is needed to control blood sugar. This type of diabetes is fatal without treatment using exogenous insulin. Glucose monitoring is necessary one to four times each day. The patient's intake of carbohydrates is controlled. Exercise is prescribed.

Type 2 Diabetes
Type 2 diabetes is more common in older adults, and the incidence increases with age. The disease used to be called adult-onset diabetes; however, the incidence of type 2 diabetes is increasing in children due increasing rates of obesity. In type 2 diabetes, the pancreas does not produce sufficient insulin or the body cannot efficiently use the insulin produced by the pancreas. This is called insulin resistance. The disease has a slow onset. It is associated with obesity. Nonketonic hyperglycemia may occur in individuals with the disease. Ketoacidosis is not common. The development of type 2 diabetes may be prevented or slowed by eating a proper diet and exercising. Type 2 diabetes is a chronic disease, and there is no known cure. Treatment is aimed at reducing mortality and morbidity and preserving quality of life. The disease is treated by diet and exercise. Oral medications are available.

Hyperglycemia
Hyperglycemia is a condition in which the serum glucose is elevated to 180 mg/dL or higher. However, symptoms may not be evident until serum glucose reaches 270 mg/dL or higher. The most common cause of hyperglycemia is diabetes mellitus, but the condition may also result from chronic pancreatitis, acromegaly, Cushing's syndrome, and adverse reactions to certain drugs (furosemide, glucocorticoids, growth hormone, oral contraceptives, and thiazides). Symptoms of hyperglycemia are similar to

those that occur with chronic diabetes. Symptoms include ketoacidosis, polyuria, polydipsia, polyphagia, weight loss, and encephalopathy. Stress-related hyperglycemia may occur after stroke and myocardial infarction and increases the risk of mortality. Physiological stress associated with infection may also increase glucose levels. Hyperglycemia can be treated with insulin and by addressing the underlying cause.

Hypoglycemia

Acute hypoglycemia (hyperinsulinism) may result from a number of conditions. Pancreatic islet tumors and hyperplasia increase insulin production, which decreases blood sugar. The use of insulin to control diabetes mellitus may cause an increase in blood sugar. Hyperinsulinism can cause damage to the central nervous system and cardiopulmonary system. Causes of acute hypoglycemia include genetic defects in chromosome 11 (short arm); severe infections (gram-negative sepsis and endotoxic shock, for example); toxic ingestion of alcohol or drugs (such as salicylates); too much insulin for body needs; and too little food or excessive exercise. Symptoms include blood glucose level less than 50 to 60 mg/dL, seizures, altered consciousness, lethargy, loss of appetite, vomiting, myoclonus, respiratory distress, diaphoresis, hypothermia, cyanosis, diaphoresis, tremor, tachycardia, palpitation, hunger, and anxiety.

Treatment depends on underlying cause and includes glucose or glucagon administration to elevate blood glucose levels, diazoxide (Hyperstat) to inhibit release of insulin, and somatostatin (Sandostatin) to suppress insulin production.

Ketoacidosis

Ketoacidosis is a complication of diabetes mellitus. Because of an insufficient production of insulin, glucose is unavailable for metabolism. As a result, fat is broken down as an alternate fuel source. Glycerol in both fat cells and the liver is converted to ketone bodies (beta-hydroxybutyrate, acetoacetic, and acetone), which are then used for cellular metabolism. Fat is a less efficient fuel than glucose. The excess ketone bodies are excreted in the urine (ketonuria) or in exhalations. The ketone bodies lower serum pH, leading to ketoacidosis. Symptoms include Kussmaul respirations (hyperventilation to eliminate buildup of carbon dioxide), fluid imbalance (resulting in dehydration and diuresis with excess thirst), cardiac arrhythmias (sometimes resulting in cardiac arrest), and hyperglycemia (blood glucose 300–800 mg/dL). Treatment includes insulin therapy by continuous infusion, rehydration, and electrolyte replacement.

Insulin Types

There are different types of insulin with varying onsets of action. *Insulin* is used to metabolize glucose in individuals whose pancreases do not produce insulin. People with diabetes may need to take a combination of insulin types. Duration of action may vary according to the individual's metabolism, intake, and level of activity: Humalog (Lispro H) is a fast-acting insulin with a short duration. It acts within 5 to15 minutes after administration, peaks within 45 to 90 minutes, and lasts 3 to 4 hours. Regular (R) is a relatively fast-acting (30 minutes) insulin that peaks in 2 to 5 hours and last 5 to 8 hours. NPH (N) or Lente (L) insulin is intermediate-acting. It acts in 1 to 3 hours after administration, peaks at 6 to12 hours, and lasts 16 to 24 hours. Ultralente (U) is long-acting insulin that acts in 4 to 6 hours, peaks at 8 to 20 hours, and lasts 24 to 28 hours. Combined NPH/Regular (70/30 or 50/50) acts in 30 minutes, peaks in 7 to 12 hours, and lasts 16 to 24 hours.

Thermoregulation

Thermoregulation is less stable in older adults, so hypothermia and malignant hyperthermia may occur more readily. Production of heat decreases, and heat loss increases. The temperature-regulating mechanism of the hypothalamus may reset the internal temperature control at a lower level. Older adults lose thermoreceptors in the skin, so they may have a delayed response to heat or cold. Older adults lose muscle mass and subcutaneous fat and the skin gets thinner. Therefore, they are less insulated against cold and have decreased heat radiation. Older adults may feel cold and chill easily. They may need to dress more warmly or increase the temperature of the room. Conversely, if a patient's temperature rises, the heart rate increases to increase heat radiation; this may put stress on a weak heart. The older patient is especially vulnerable to heat exhaustion or heat stroke in temperatures higher than 90 degrees Fahrenheit with high humidity. Hypothermia (a core temperature less than 94° F) may be indicated by shivering and muscle pain. If the hypothermia persists, alterations in consciousness occur followed by coma, cyanosis, and death.

Thyroid

Hypothyroidism

Hypothyroidism is a condition in which the thyroid produces inadequate amounts of thyroid hormones. The condition may range from mild to severe. There are a number of causes: chronic lymphocytic thyroiditis (Hashimoto's thyroiditis); excessive treatment for hyperthyroidism; atrophy of the thyroid gland; medications, such as lithium and iodine compounds; radiation to the area of the thyroid; diseases that affect the thyroid, such as scleroderma; and iodine imbalances. Signs and symptoms include chronic fatigue, menstrual disturbances, hoarseness, subnormal temperature, low pulse rate, weight gain, thinning hair, and thickening skin. Some dementia may occur in advanced cases. Clinical findings may include increased cholesterol levels with associated atherosclerosis and coronary artery disease. Myxedema may occur. Signs and symptoms include changes in respiration with

hypoventilation and CO_2 retention resulting in coma. Treatment involves hormone replacement with synthetic levothyroxine (Synthroid) based on thyroid-stimulating hormone (TSH) levels. However, this increases the oxygen requirements of the body, necessitating careful monitoring of cardiac status to avoid myocardial infarction while establishing the normal hormone levels.

Hyperthyroidism

Hyperthyroidism (thyrotoxicosis) is a condition in which excessive amounts of thyroid hormones are produced by the thyroid gland. This occurs as a result of abnormal stimulation of the thyroid gland by immunoglobulins. Other causes include thyroiditis (inflammation of the thyroid) and excessive amounts of thyroid medication. Symptoms vary and may be nonspecific, especially in the elderly. Symptoms include hyperexcitability, tachycardia, atrial fibrillation, increased systolic (but not diastolic) blood pressure, poor heat tolerance, flushed skin, diaphoresis, dry skin, pruritis (especially in the elderly), hand tremor, progressive muscular weakness, exophthalmos (bulging eyes), and increased appetite and food intake with weight loss. Treatment involves a series of actions. Radioactive iodine is administered to destroy the thyroid gland. Propranolol may be used to prevent thyroid storm. Thyroid hormones are given for resultant hypothyroidism. Antithyroid medications, such as Propacil or Tapazole, are administered to block the conversion of thyroxine (T4) to triiodothyronine (T3). The thyroid is surgically removed if the patient cannot tolerate other treatments or if there is a large goiter involved. One-sixth of the thyroid is usually left in place.

Thyrotoxic Storm

A thyrotoxic storm is a severe form of hyperthyroidism. A toxic storm is precipitated by stress. Toxic storms occur in individuals with untreated or inadequately treated hyperthyroidism. If not treated promptly, the condition is fatal. The incidence of the condition has decreased with the advent of antithyroid medications, but it may still occur in medical emergencies or during pregnancy. Signs and symptoms include temperature increase to 38.5 degrees Celsius or more; tachycardia; atrial fibrillation; heart failure; gastrointestinal disorders (such as nausea, vomiting, diarrhea, and abdominal discomfort); and altered mental status (delirium progressing to coma). Diagnostic findings include increased T3 uptake and decreased thyroid-stimulating hormone (TSH). Treatment includes controlling the production of thyroid hormone through the use of antithyroid medications (such as propylthiouracil and methimazole), inhibiting the release of thyroid hormone with iodine therapy (or lithium), and controlling peripheral activity of thyroid hormone with propranolol. In addition, treatment may include fluid and electrolyte replacement, administration of glucocorticoids (such as dexamethasone), the use of cooling blankets, and the administration of antiarrhythmics and anticoagulants.

Electrolyte Imbalances

Sodium
The normal sodium level is 135 to 145 mEq/L. Hyponatremia and hypernatremia are sodium electrolyte imbalances.

- Hyponatremia is defined as a sodium level of less than 135 mEq/L. The condition may result from an insufficient intake of sodium or an abnormal loss of sodium through diarrhea, vomiting, and nasogastric suctioning. It can occur following severe burns and as a result of fever and illnesses such as syndrome of inappropriate antidiuretic hormone secretion (SIADH) and ketoacidosis. Symptoms vary and may include irritability, lethargy, and alterations in consciousness. Cerebral edema can lead to seizures and coma. Dyspnea

can lead to respiratory failure. Treatment involves identifying and treating the underlying cause and providing sodium replacement.
- Hypernatremia is defined as a sodium level of greater than 145 mEq/L. Hypernatremia may occur as a result of renal disease, diabetes insipidus, or fluid depletion. Signs and symptoms of hypernatremia include irritability, lethargy, confusion, coma, seizures, flushing, muscle weakness and spasms, and thirst. Treatment includes identification and treatment of the underlying cause and intravenous fluid replacement.

Potassium

Hypokalemia
Hypokalemia is an abnormally low potassium level. Potassium is the primary electrolyte in intracellular fluid. Approximately 98 percent of the potassium in the body is found inside cells, and only 2 percent is found in the extracellular fluid. Potassium affects the activity of the skeletal and cardiac muscles. Potassium level is dependent on renal functioning, because 80 percent is excreted in urine and 20 percent in feces and sweat. The normal potassium level is 3.5 to 5.5 mEq/L. In hypokalemia, the level of potassium is less than 3.5 mEq/L. Hypokalemia may be caused by loss of potassium through diarrhea, vomiting, gastric suction, diuresis, alkalosis, decreased potassium intake with starvation, and nephritis. Signs and symptoms of hypokalemia include lethargy, weakness, nausea, vomiting, paresthesia, dysrhythmia, premature ventricular contractions (PVCs), flattened T waves, muscle cramps with hyporeflexia, hypotension, and tetany. Treatment includes the identification of the underlying cause of the disorder and potassium replacement.

Hyperkalemia
Hyperkalemia is an abnormally high level of potassium (greater than 5.5 mEq/L).

Hyperkalemia may be caused by renal disease, adrenal insufficiency, metabolic acidosis, severe dehydration, burns, hemolysis, and trauma. The disorder rarely occurs without renal disease but may be induced by treatment (such as nonsteroidal anti-inflammatory drugs [NSAIDs] and potassium-sparing diuretics). Untreated renal disease results in reduced excretion of potassium. Individuals with Addison's disease and a deficiency of adrenal hormones may suffer a sodium loss that results in potassium retention. The primary symptoms relate to the effect on the cardiac muscle. Signs and symptoms are as follows: ventricular arrhythmias leading to cardiac and respiratory arrest, weakness with ascending paralysis and hyperreflexia, diarrhea, and increasing mental confusion. Treatment includes identification of the underlying cause, discontinuation of sources of excess potassium, administration of calcium gluconate to decrease cardiac effects, administration of sodium bicarbonate (to shift potassium into the cells temporarily), administration of insulin and hypertonic dextrose (to shift potassium into the cells temporarily), use of cation exchange resin (Kayexalate) (to decrease potassium), and peritoneal dialysis or hemodialysis.

Hypocalcemia and Hypercalcemia

One percent of the calcium in the body is in the serum. Serum calcium is important for transmitting nerve impulses and regulating muscle contraction and relaxation. Calcium activates enzymes that stimulate chemical reactions, and it plays a role in blood clotting. The normal calcium level is 1.15 to 1.34 mg/dL. In hypocalcemia, the level is less than 1.15 mg/dL. In hypercalcemia, the level is greater than 1.34 mg/dL.

- Hypocalcemia may be caused by hypoparathyroidism. It also occurs after thyroid and parathyroid surgery and as a result of pancreatitis, renal failure, inadequate vitamin D intake, alkalosis, magnesium deficiency and low serum albumin. Signs and symptoms include tetany, tingling, seizures, altered mental status, and ventricular tachycardia. Treatment includes calcium replacement and vitamin D supplementation.

- Hypercalcemia may be caused by acidosis, kidney disease, hyperparathyroidism, prolonged immobilization, and malignancies. A hypercalcemic crisis carries a 50 percent mortality rate. Signs and symptoms include muscle weakness with hypotonicity, anorexia, nausea, vomiting, constipation, bradycardia, and cardiac arrest. Treatment includes identification and treatment of the underlying cause and administration of loop diuretics and IV fluids.

Hypophosphatemi and Hyperphosphatemia

Phosphorus, or phosphate (PO_4), is necessary for neuromuscular and red blood cell function and for the maintenance of acid-base balance. Phosphorus provides structure for teeth and bones. About 85 percent is in the bones, 14 percent in soft tissue, and less than 1 percent in extracellular fluid. The normal level of phosphorus is 2.4 to 4.5 mEq/L. In hypophosphatemia, the phosphorus level is less than 2.4 mEq/L. In hyperphosphatemia, the level is greater than 4.5 mEq/L.

- Hypophosphatemia occurs in the following situations: severe protein-calorie malnutrition; excessive use of antacids containing magnesium, calcium, or aluminum; hyperventilation; severe burn injuries; and diabetic ketoacidosis. Signs and symptoms include irritability, tremors, seizures, coma, hemolytic anemia, decreased myocardial function, and respiratory failure. Treatment involves identification of the underlying cause and phosphorus replacement.

- Hyperphosphatemia occurs in the following situations: renal failure, hypoparathyroidism, excessive intake of phosphate, neoplastic disease, diabetic ketoacidosis, muscle necrosis, and chemotherapy. Signs and symptoms include tachycardia, muscle cramping, hyperreflexia, tetany, nausea, and diarrhea. Treatment involves identification of the underlying cause, correction of hypocalcemia, and provision of antacids and dialysis.

Hypomagnesemia and Hypermagnesemia
Magnesium (Mg) is the second most common intracellular electrolyte (after potassium). Magnesium activates many intracellular enzyme systems. It is important for carbohydrate and protein metabolism, neuromuscular function, and cardiovascular function.

Magnesium produces vasodilation and directly affects the peripheral arterial system. The normal level of magnesium is 1.4 mEq/L. In hypomagnesemia, magnesium level is less than 1.4 mEq/L. In hypermagnesemia, magnesium level is greater than 1.4 mEq/L.

- Hypomagnesemia occurs in the following situations: chronic diarrhea, chronic renal disease, chronic pancreatitis, excessive diuretic or laxative use, hyperthyroidism, hypoparathyroidism, severe burn injuries, and diaphoresis. Signs and symptoms include neuromuscular excitability/tetany, mental confusion, headaches, dizziness, seizure, coma, tachycardia with ventricular arrhythmia, and respiratory depression. Treatment involves identification of the underlying cause and magnesium replacement.
- Hypermagnesemia occurs in the following situations: renal failure or inadequate renal function, diabetic ketoacidosis, hypothyroidism, and Addison's disease. Signs and symptoms include muscle weakness, seizures, dysphagia with decreased gag reflex, and tachycardia with

hypotension. Treatment includes identification of the underlying cause, intravenous hydration with calcium, and dialysis.

Acidosis

Metabolic Acidosis
Metabolic acidosis is an increase in the acidity of the plasma. It involves a disruption of the body's acid-base balance. A number of different disorders can lead to metabolic acidosis. These include kidney failure, diabetic ketoacidosis, starvation, and shock. In addition, the disorder can be caused by ingesting certain toxic substances (such as antifreeze and large amounts of aspirin). Metabolic acidosis may result in shock or death. Signs and symptoms of this disorder include rapid breathing, mental confusion, lethargy, arrhythmia, nausea, vomiting, and abdominal pain. The condition can be a mild, chronic disorder in some cases. Diagnostic tests include arterial blood gas, metabolic panel, and blood count. Treatment includes addressing the underlying cause. Bicarbonate may be administered. This treatment can decrease the blood's acidity.

Respiratory Acidosis
Respiratory acidosis is an abnormal drop in the pH level of the blood. This condition occurs because of reduced ventilation of the alveoli. This leads to a rapid increase in the concentration of carbon dioxide in the arteries. The body fluids become increasingly acidic. The condition can be acute or chronic. In the acute form, the carbon dioxide increases too rapidly for the kidneys to compensate. In the chronic form, respiratory acidosis takes place over a longer period, allowing the kidneys time to compensate. In chronic respiratory acidosis, the kidneys produce chemicals to control the acid-base balance. Causes of respiratory acidosis include asthma and chronic obstructive pulmonary disease, skeletal disorders that prevent the lungs from filling efficiently, nerve disorders that interfere with lung

inflation or deflation, obesity, and ingestion of certain drugs (such as narcotics and benzodiazepines). Signs and symptoms include mental confusion, lethargy, and shortness of breath. Diagnostic techniques include tests of pulmonary function, chest x-ray, computed tomography (CT) scan, and arterial blood gas. Treatment includes bronchodilator medications, noninvasive positive-pressure ventilation, mechanical ventilation, and oxygen administration.

Metabolic Alkalosis

Metabolic alkalosis is a disorder involving an abnormally elevated blood pH. The disorder can be caused by excessive vomiting over a prolonged period of time, severe dehydration, the ingestion of alkali substances, and the administration of diuretics. Endocrine disorders (such as Cushing's syndrome) can also cause metabolic alkalosis. Hypokalemia and hypocalcemia may accompany metabolic alkalosis. Metabolic alkalosis may indicate dysfunction of a major organ. Symptoms include slow breathing, cyanosis, dizziness, mental confusion, tremors, muscle cramping, tetany, tachycardia, arrhythmia, nausea, vomiting, loss of appetite, and compensatory hypoventilation. Metabolic alkalosis is diagnosed based on the patient's symptoms. The disorder is confirmed with laboratory tests. A blood pH of more than 7.45 is confirmative. The levels of other components of the blood (potassium, chloride, and sodium, for example) are below normal. Serum bicarbonate level is elevated. The aim of treatment is to restore the acid-base balance. Treatment includes the administration of normal saline and potassium chloride. Medication may be administered to regulate blood pressure and heart rate. The underlying condition must be treated.

Respiratory Alkalosis

Respiratory alkalosis is a disorder in which the blood contains abnormally low levels of carbon dioxide. Respiratory alkalosis occurs as a result of alveolar hyperventilation.

Respiratory alkalosis may be acute or chronic. In the chronic state, the body compensates and reduces the effect of alkalosis. Respiratory alkalosis has a number of causes, including hyperventilation, anxiety, hysteria, fever, stroke, and use of certain drugs (such as doxapram). Caffeine and aspirin overdose can also cause this disorder. Signs and symptoms include dizziness, light-headedness, and numbness in the extremities. Seizures may occur in severe cases, but this is extremely uncommon. Diagnosis is based on arterial blood gas, chest x-ray, and pulmonary function tests. Treatment for respiratory alkalosis depends on the cause of the disorder. The underlying condition must be addressed. A rebreathing mask may be used

Advanced Clinical Practice

Postmenopausal Changes

The female reproduction system undergoes a number of <u>postmenopausal changes</u>. The ovaries still produce some hormones, but by late postmenopause, the production of estrogen has dropped by 80 percent and progesterone by 60 percent. Mental functioning may be affected. The decrease in estrogen levels may result in cognitive decline, insomnia, and depression. The skin becomes thinner and loses collagen. Hair follicles become dry. Bones lose calcium and become more porous. As connective tissue is lost, breasts begin to droop. The bladder starts to function less efficiently. The ovaries atrophy. The uterus shrinks to about 50 percent of its original size and may not be palpable in women older than age 75. The cervix may retract. The vagina becomes shorter. The walls of the vagina become thinner and lose elasticity and lubrication; this may result in painful sexual intercourse. The vaginal fluid becomes more alkaline. The labia majora shrink and separate. This exposes the inner structures and increases the risk of infection.

HIV

Human immunodeficiency virus, commonly referred to as HIV, is a slow-acting retrovirus of the genus lentivirus. The virus is spread through contact with infected body fluids. HIV attacks the body by binding with cells that have CD4 receptors. These are primarily CD4+ T cells and other cells of the immune system. The virus enters the cells and starts replicating. The virus destroys the host cells in a number of ways: The virus disrupts the cell membrane when large numbers of viral cells push through the cell membrane. Cell function is disrupted when large numbers of viral cells accumulate within a host cell. Syncytia are formed when HIV-infected host cells fuse with nearby cells. This process creates giant cells and facilitates the spread of the virus. The virus also signals uninfected cells to self-destruct. The binding of HIV cells to host cell membranes causes the host cell to be targeted by killer T cells as part of the immune response.

AIDS

Acquired immunodeficiency syndrome (AIDS) is caused by HIV. Individuals older than age 50 comprise the fastest growing group of AIDS patients. As people age and acquire other diseases in addition to AIDS, management becomes complicated. The diagnostic criteria for AIDS include HIV infection; a CD4 count of greater than 200 cells/mm^3; and AIDS-defining conditions, such as opportunistic infections (cytomegalovirus, tuberculosis), wasting syndrome, neoplasms (Kaposi's sarcoma), or AIDS dementia complex. Because of the wide range of AIDS-defining conditions, the patient may present with many types of symptoms. However, more than half of patients exhibit fever, lymphadenopathy, pharyngitis, rash, and myalgia/arthralgia. It is important to review the following when making a diagnosis: CD4 counts (to determine immune status), white blood cell count and differential (for signs of infection), cultures (to help identify any infective agents), and complete blood count (to evaluate for signs of bleeding or thrombocytopenia). Treatment is designed to cure or manage opportunistic conditions and control the underlying HIV infection. Highly active antiretroviral therapy (HAART) is administered. Three or more drugs are used concurrently.

Successive Stages of Alzheimer's Disease

Alzheimer's disease may be staged in a number of ways. There is no specific test for Alzheimer's disease. Staging is based on a combination of a physical examination, history (often provided by family or caregivers), and mental assessment. The seven-stage classification system (developed by Barry Reisberg, MD) is used by the Alzheimer's Association.

- Stage 1 is preclinical. There is no evident impairment, although slight changes may be occurring within the brain.
- Stage 2 involves very mild cognitive decline. Patients may misplace items and forget thoughts or words. However, impairment is not usually noticeable to others or evident on medical examination.
- Stage 3 is defined by mild, early-stage cognitive decline with short-term memory loss and problems with reading retention and name recall. The patient may have trouble handling money, planning, and organizing. The patient may also misplace items of value.
- Stage 4 of Alzheimer's disease is defined by moderate cognitive decline with decreased knowledge of current affairs and/or family history. The patient exhibits social withdrawal and has difficulty with complex tasks. This stage is more easily recognized on examination and may persist for 2 to 10 years. During this stage, the patient may be able to manage most activities of daily living and hygiene.
- Stage 5 is defined by moderately severe cognitive decline. Brain changes are evident; the cerebral cortex and hippocampus shrink and the ventricles enlarge. Patients are obviously confused and disoriented regarding date, time, and place. Patients may have difficulty using and/or understanding speech and managing activities of daily living. They may forget their address and telephone number. Individuals at this stage of the disease may dress inappropriately, forget to eat and lose weight, or eat a poor diet. They may

be unable to do simple math, such as counting backward by twos.

- Stage 6 of Alzheimer's disease is defined by moderately severe cognitive decline; the brain continues to shrink and neurons die. Patients are profoundly confused and unable to care for themselves. Individuals at this stage may undergo profound personality changes. Patients may confuse fantasy and reality. They may fail to recognize family members and experience difficulty toileting. Patients at this stage of the disease tend to pace obsessively or wander away. Patients may exhibit sundowner's syndrome, a disruption of the waking/sleeping cycle. Individuals with this syndrome tend to become restless and wander about at night. Patients may develop obsessive behaviors, such as tearing items, pulling at the hair, or wringing of the hands. This stage (with stage 7) may be prolonged, lasting one to five years.
- Stage 7 is defined by very severe cognitive decline. During this stage, most patients are wheelchair bound or bed bound. Most patients lose the ability to speak beyond a few words. They exhibit urinary and bowel incontinence and may be unable to sit unsupported or hold their head up. They choke easily and have increased weakness and rigidity of muscles.

Non-Alzheimer's Dementias

The following are non-Alzheimer's dementias:

- Creutzfeldt-Jakob disease is a rapidly progressing dementia causing memory impairments, behavioral changes, and loss of coordination.
- Dementia with Lewy bodies involves a cognitive and physical decline similar to Alzheimer's disease, but symptoms may fluctuate frequently. This form of

- 47 -

dementia may involve visual hallucinations, muscle rigidity, and tremors.

- Frontotemporal dementia may cause marked changes in personality and behavior. The dementia is characterized by difficulty using and understanding language.
- Mixed dementia is a combination of Alzheimer's and another type of dementia. Symptoms of the dementias interact.
- Normal-pressure hydrocephalus is characterized by ataxia, memory loss, and urinary incontinence.
- Parkinson's dementia may involve impairments in the following domains: making decisions, concentrating, learning new material, understanding complex language, and sequencing. The patient may be inflexible and exhibit short- or long-term memory loss.
- Vascular dementia has symptoms similar to Alzheimer's disease, but memory loss may be less pronounced.

Delirium

Delirium is an acute, sudden change in consciousness. It is characterized by reduced ability to focus or sustain attention, language and memory impairment, disorientation, confusion, audiovisual hallucinations, sleep disturbance, and psychomotor activity disorder. The symptoms of delirium fluctuate. Delirium occurs in 10 to 40 percent of hospitalized older adults and in about 80 percent of terminally ill patients. Delirium may result from the use of certain drugs (such as anticholinergics) and from numerous conditions including infection, hypoxia, trauma, dementia, depression, vision and hearing loss, surgery, alcoholism, untreated pain, fluid/electrolyte imbalance, and malnutrition. Delirium increases the risk of morbidity and death, especially if untreated. Diagnosis is based on patient interview and history and chart review. Asking the patient

to count backward from 20 to 1 and spell his or her first name backward can identify an attention deficit. Treatment includes decreasing the dosage of hypnotics and psychotropics. Medications administered to reduce symptoms include trazodone, lorazepam, and haloperidol.

Sleep Disorders

Older adults often take longer to fall asleep at night and awaken more frequently than younger adults. They also sleep more often during the day. Approximately 50 percent of older adults have insomnia, while 65 to 70 percent have combined sleep disorders. Sleep disorders include sleep apnea, insomnia, circadian rhythm disorders, and sleep-related movement disorders. Patients may not report sleep disorders but may present with vague complaints of feeling tired, lethargic, and depressed. Sleep disorders in older adults may be related to pain; incontinence; urinary frequency; obesity; neurodegenerative diseases; dyspnea; depression; anxiety disorders; bereavement; poor sleep habits; medications (such as benzodiazepines, antidepressants, diuretics, anti-Parkinson drugs, and anticonvulsants); caffeine; and alcohol. An overnight sleep study utilizing polysomnography (PSG) and sleep diaries may aid diagnosis. Treatment includes bright-light therapy in the evening to keep the individual awake and medication to induce sleep. The patient may be advised to keep the bedroom dark at night, keep set times for sleeping and arising, avoid excessive napping, eliminate caffeine, reduce noise at night, and increase daytime activity. Treatment for restless legs syndrome or sleep apnea may be required.

Strokes

Ischemic Stroke
Strokes result when there is interruption of the blood flow to an area of the brain. The two primary types are ischemic and hemorrhagic. Approximately 80 percent are

ischemic strokes, resulting from blockage of an artery supplying the brain. *Thrombosis* is the formation of a blood clot in a blood vessel. Thrombosis in a large artery, usually resulting from atherosclerosis, may block circulation to a large area of the brain. This condition occurs most frequently in the elderly and may occur suddenly or after a transient ischemic attack. A lacunar infarct (penetrating thrombosis in a small artery) is most common in those with diabetes mellitus and/or hypertension. An *embolism* (wandering blood clot) passes through the circulatory system and lodges in the brain, most commonly in the left middle cerebral artery. A cardiogenic embolism results from cardiac arrhythmia or surgery. An embolism usually has a sudden onset and often occurs with no warning signs. A cryptogenic stroke has no identifiable cause.

Hemorrhagic Stroke

Approximately 20 percent of strokes are hemorrhagic. Hemorrhagic strokes result from a ruptured cerebral artery. They cause an interruption in the supply of oxygen and nutrients. In addition, they cause edema, which results in widespread pressure and damage. An intracerebral hemorrhage involves bleeding from an artery in the central lobes, basal ganglia, pons, or cerebellum into the brain matter. Intracerebral hemorrhage may result from atherosclerotic degenerative changes, hypertension, brain tumors, anticoagulation therapy, or use of some illicit drugs, such as crack and cocaine. Onset is often sudden and the condition may be fatal. An intracranial aneurysm occurs in ballooning cerebral artery ruptures, most commonly at the circle of Willis. An *arteriovenous malformation* (AVM) is a tangle of dilated arteries and veins without a capillary bed. This is a congenital abnormality. Rupture of AVMs is a cause of stroke in young adults. A *subarachnoid hemorrhage* is bleeding in the space between the meninges and brain. It results from aneurysm, AVM, or trauma. This type of hemorrhage compresses brain tissue.

Brain Strokes

Strokes most frequently occur in the *right* or *left hemisphere*. The exact location and the extent of brain damage affect the presenting symptoms. If the frontal area on either side of the brain is involved, memory and learning deficits are usually evident. Some symptoms are unique to specific areas and help to identify the area involved.

- Right Hemisphere: A stroke in the right hemisphere results in paralysis or paresis on the left side and a left visual field deficit that may cause spatial and perceptual disturbances. People with this type of damage may have difficulty judging distance. Fine motor skills may be adversely affected, resulting in trouble dressing or handling tools. People may become impulsive and exhibit poor judgment, often denying any impairment. Left-sided neglect (lack of perception of things on the left side) may be evident. Depression, short-term memory loss, and difficulty following directions are often evident. Language skills usually remain intact.
- Left-hemisphere stroke: results in paralysis or paresis on the right side and a right visual field deficit. Depression is common and people often behave in a slow, cautious manner, requiring repeated instruction and reinforcement for simple tasks. Short-term memory loss and difficulty learning new material or understanding generalizations is common. Difficulty with mathematics, reading, writing, and reasoning may be evident. Aphasia (expressive, receptive, or global) is common.
- A brain-stem stroke frequently causes death because the brain stem controls respiration and cardiac function. Individuals who survive may have a number of problems, including respiratory and cardiac abnormalities. Strokes may involve

- 49 -

motor impairment, sensory impairment, or both.

- The cerebellum controls balance and coordination. Strokes in the cerebellum are rare but may result in ataxia, nausea, vomiting, headaches, and dizziness or vertigo.

Parkinson's Disease

Parkinson's disease (PD) is an extrapyramidal movement motor system disorder. It results from loss of brain cells that produce dopamine. Typical symptoms include tremor in the face and extremities, rigidity, bradykinesia, akinesia, poor posture, and lack of balance and coordination. These symptoms cause increasing problems with mobility, speaking, and swallowing. Some individuals with Parkinson's disease may suffer depression, mood changes, and dementia. Unilateral tremors in an upper extremity are usually evident. Diagnosis methods include the cogwheel rigidity test (passive range of motion causes an increase in muscle tone and ratchetlike movements in the affected extremity), a physical and neurological examination, and a complete medical history.

Treatment includes administration of dopaminergic drugs (levodopa, amantadine, and carbidopa) and anticholinergic drugs (trihexyphenidyl and benztropine). In cases of drug-induced Parkinson's, the drugs causing the disorder must be discontinued. Drug therapy tends to decrease in efficacy over time, and symptoms may worsen. Discontinuing the drugs for one week may cause the symptoms to worsen initially, but functioning may improve when drugs are reintroduced.

Mental Health

Mental Retardation

Older adults with mental retardation (MR) or a developmental disorder now have a life expectancy of approximately 66 years. However, the life expectancy of younger adults with MR is approximately 76 years. Adults with MR pose challenges for health-care providers. The most common cause of mental retardation is Down syndrome. Older adults with MR often have associated medical conditions. Vision impairment related to cataracts, nystagmus, hyperplasia, corneal abnormalities, and refractive disorders are very common in this population and often remain uncorrected. Severe mental retardation is positively correlated with severity of ocular disorders. About 50 percent of individuals older than age 50 with Down syndrome have cataracts. Hearing loss is very common in individuals with Down syndrome (70 percent of individuals age 59 and under). Poor dental care in adults with MR is common as these individuals may not care for their teeth properly. All people with mental retardation should have a complete dental exam.

Thyroid dysfunction

Thyroid dysfunction is common in older adults with MR and is often not diagnosed. Therefore, all people with mental retardation should have their thyroid tested.

Obesity

Approximately 48 percent of mentally retarded individuals are *obese*, and this puts them at increased risk for cardiovascular disease. *Osteoporosis* is common in people older than age 50 often because of poor diet and immobility. It may be associated with osteoarthritis.

Mental health disorders are more common among individuals with MR than among individuals in the general population. These disorders include mood disorders (such as bipolar disorder) and schizophrenia. Behavioral disorders (such as aggression, agitation, and sleep disturbances) are also more common among individuals with MR. Patients may engage in self-injurious behavior. By age 65, approximately 20 percent of individuals with non–Down syndrome mental retardation have dementia, but this number increases to 52 percent by age 88. Individuals with Down syndrome exhibit signs of dementia earlier, with about 42 percent exhibiting dementia by age 50.

Grief

Grief is a normal response to loss. Older adults may have to face the loss of their spouse, family, income, status, health, mobility, home, and independence. Mourning is the public expression of grief, and bereavement is the time period of mourning. There are three primary types of grief: *acute, anticipatory, and chronic. Acute grief* is immediate and occurs in response to some type of loss. It may be expressed as sadness, anger, fear, and anxiety.

Anticipatory grief

Anticipatory grief occurs when a loss is feared. For example, anticipatory grief may occur when the death of a spouse is impending. *Chronic* grief occurs when people are not able to come to terms with a loss so that grieving and mourning are prolonged, sometimes for years. People experiencing chronic grief may develop anorexia, insomnia, panic attacks, and self-destructive behaviors (alcohol and substance abuse). They may even contemplate or commit suicide. Chronic grief poses a serious risk to people and should be treated in the same way as depression with antidepressants, psychological evaluation, and counseling.

Depression

Depression affects about 19 percent of adults older than age 55. Further, it affects approximately 37 percent of older adults who have comorbid conditions. Older adults have the highest rate of suicide and are at risk. Depression is associated with conditions that decrease quality of life, such as heart disease, neuromuscular disease, arthritis, cancer, diabetes, Huntington's disease, stroke, and diabetes. Some drugs (diuretics, Parkinson's drugs, estrogen, corticosteroids, cimetidine, hydralazine, propranolol, digitalis, and indomethacin, for example) may also

precipitate depression. Depressed patients experience mood changes, sadness, loss of interest in usual activities, fatigue, appetite changes, weight fluctuations, anxiety, and sleep disturbance. Depression often goes undiagnosed, so screening for at-risk individuals should be performed routinely. Treatment includes TCAs and selective serotonin reuptake inhibitors (SSRIs). SSRIs have fewer side effects and are less likely to cause death with an overdose. Older adults may take longer to respond to medication than younger adults. Treatment includes counseling, addressing the underlying cause, and instituting an exercise program.

Schizophrena

Schizophrenia is a related group of psychiatric illnesses. The subtypes of the disorder include paranoid, disorganized, catatonic, undifferentiated, and residual. Symptoms vary widely but include positive symptoms and negative symptoms. Positive symptoms include delusions and hallucinations, and negative symptoms include flat affect and lack of motivation. Comorbidities, such as obsessive-compulsive disorder, depression, and substance abuse are common. Patients may have suicidal tendencies. In older adults, psychosis is often less severe. However, some cognitive impairment is common at all ages and is a persistent problem with chronic schizophrenia. There are approximately 300,000 older adult schizophrenics in the United States; about two-thirds of these are in nursing homes. However, only 15,000 are in psychiatric hospitals, suggesting that cognitive impairment is the bigger problem in older adults. Treatment for schizophrenia includes typical antipsychotics (chlorpromazine, haloperidol, loxapine) and atypical antipsychotics (olanzapine, clozapine, risperidone). Atypical antipsychotics are more effective at reducing negative symptoms. All medications are associated with significant side effects, including tardive dyskinesia, but atypical antipsychotics have fewer side effects.

Studies suggest that atypical antipsychotics may be better tolerated by older adults.

Bipolar disorder

Bipolar disorder is an affective disorder characterized by mood swings ranging from depression to mania. The disorder includes several subtypes: bipolar I, bipolar II, cyclothymia, rapid cycling, and mixed state. Comorbid conditions include substance abuse, thyroid disorders, suicidal tendencies, obsessive-compulsive disorder, post-traumatic stress disorder, and dementia. Individuals with late-onset bipolar disorder (occurring after the age of 50) tend to exhibit less severe symptoms than those with early onset bipolar disorder. Symptoms include severe mania, hypomania, normal mood, mild to moderate depression, and severe depression. Symptoms may be triggered by environmental factors, such as medication, stress, substance abuse, sleep disorders, and changes of season. The disorder is treated by various medications (mood stabilizers, anticonvulsants, and atypical antipsychotics). Antidepressants are contraindicated. Treatment with one drug (mood stabilizer) is the goal for older adults because of the potential for adverse effects and drug interactions. Electroshock treatment is effective for older adults in the depressed state. The half-life of drugs is increased in older adults because of reduced renal clearance, so it is often necessary to administer lower doses. Careful monitoring is necessary.

Anxiety disorders

Anxiety disorders affect approximately 11 percent of individuals older than age 50. Generalized anxiety disorder and panic disorder are classified as anxiety disorders.

Generalized anxiety disorder

Generalized anxiety disorder is usually a chronic condition that manifests early in life. Symptoms include chronic worry, sleep disorders, restlessness, impaired concentration, fatigue, and depression (in 47%). A panic attack is an autonomic response. *Panic disorder* involves acute episodes (attacks) of tachycardia, dyspnea, diaphoresis, faintness, and weakness. In older adults, autonomic response to anxiety may be muted and the symptoms of panic attack less pronounced and more nonspecific (weak, light-headed, slight increase in pulse/respiration). Anxiety is predictive of increased cognitive impairment and lower pain tolerance. Individuals with chronic medical conditions are more likely to become anxious. During acute episodes, supportive care in a quiet environment should be provided. The nurse should remain with the patient and provide reassurance in a calm voice. The patient should be reoriented without being asked to make decisions. Long-term treatment includes deep-breathing exercises, progressive muscle relaxation, and cognitive behavioral therapy. Medications include selective serotonin reuptake inhibitors (SSRIs) and serotonin-norepinephrine reuptake inhibitors (SNRIs).

Social isolation

Social isolation is pervasive among older adults and is correlated with feelings of loneliness. The social activity of individuals decreases as they age. Family and friends die, move to nursing homes, or relocate. *Loneliness* is especially common among adults who are widowed. Surprisingly, loneliness is common among older adults living with their grown children. Social isolation and loneliness are exacerbated by disease and anxiety. Older adults often have very little social interaction and many are neglected by family and friends. Loneliness can lead to stress-related disorders (hypertension, cardiovascular disease, and diabetes mellitus, for example). Research has demonstrated that although older women tend to be more isolated than men, men suffer more acutely from loneliness than women. Loneliness appears to increase the risk of dementia associated with Alzheimer's disease. Loneliness may have a negative effect on the nervous system. Effective interventions include involving older adults in group activities that promote social interaction.

Management of Suicidal Patients

Approximately 50 percent of suicides involving older adults are associated with depression. For this reason, all depressed older patients should be assessed for suicide risk. Suicide has many possible causes, including severe depression, social isolation, situational crisis (move to nursing home), bereavement, and psychosis. The nurse should provide support without being judgmental because this may further harm the patient's self-esteem and increase the risk of another suicide attempt. Suicidal patients should be referred to a mental health professional for evaluation. Treatment for a suicide attempt depends on the type of suicide attempt. There are antidotes available for certain common drugs. For example naloxone (Narcan) is given for opiate overdose and N-acetylcysteine is administered for acetaminophen overdose. Individuals at high risk for a further suicide attempt should be hospitalized. High-risk situations include violent suicide attempt (knives, gunshots); suicide attempt with low chance of rescue; ongoing psychosis; ongoing severe depression; repeated suicide attempts; and lack of a social support system.

Substance Abuse

Substance abuse by the elderly often remains undiagnosed. However, approximately 10 to15 percent of older adults abuse alcohol and many abuse other drugs. Alcohol and drug abuse is often linked to an underlying psychiatric disorder.

Prescription drugs include narcotics and benzodiazepines. Overuse of prescription drugs, especially psychotropics, is common among older adults. Abuse of benzodiazepine may lead to an increase in falls and auto accidents. The effects of benzodiazepine are potentiated if the drug is taken with alcohol or narcotics. Patients may experience withdrawal symptoms if the medication, especially Xanax, is stopped suddenly.

Drug abusers often have multiple prescriptions from different doctors.

Nonprescription drugs include over-the-counter sleep preparations and alcohol. Alcohol may cause symptoms similar to those of depression. Individuals who abuse alcohol may develop chronic disorders (such as cirrhosis, cardiomyopathy, and neuropathy), because many alcoholics do not eat a healthy diet and suffer from B_1 deficiency. Further, alcohol brain syndrome can develop and lead to suicide. Withdrawal may cause delirium tremens and seizures.

Illicit drugs include marijuana. Older adults are less likely to use heroin or cocaine.

Inappropriate Sexual Behavior

The sexual feelings of older adults with dementia or cognitive impairment may be expressed inappropriately. These individuals may undress, masturbate, request sexual favors, use obscene language, or behave aggressively. Such inappropriate behavior may be out of character for the individual.

Inappropriate sexual behavior may be prompted by lack of inhibition and decreased reasoning ability. This behavior may be of brief duration during a phase or may persist for a prolonged period of time (months or years). In some cases, such as disrobing publicly, the person may simply be hot or need to urinate or defecate. People may relieve themselves in inappropriate places, such as a wastebasket, in response to physical need. If the individual exhibits violent sexual behavior, medication may be prescribed to try to manage it. However, in general, medication does little to prevent or lessen inappropriate behavior. Inappropriate sexual behavior is best managed by supervision. The patient may exhibit certain patterns of behavior (such as pulling at clothes) before engaging in inappropriate sexual behavior. The behavior may be prevented if the patient is distracted.

Cognitively Impaired Patients

Patients with Alzheimer's disease and cognitive impairment become easily confused. Therefore, a regular schedule should be maintained for the patient if possible. Simple choices may be overwhelming for the patient, and caregivers should avoid having the patient make unnecessary choices. Directions should involve only one or two simple steps. Clothes without zippers or buttons may be easiest for the patient and caregivers to manage. Patients may resist bathing. In this case, Comfort Bath disposable washcloths may be used; one part of the body is washed at a time. For example, the face and arms may be washed in the morning and the trunk and legs at night. If the patient wants to pace, he or she should be allowed to do so if possible. Attempting to stop the patient from pacing rarely succeeds and will cause the patient distress. It may be helpful to take the patient outside for a walk.

<u>Supportive Care</u>
Patients with Alzheimer's disease or cognitive impairment may be disruptive and difficult to manage. Caregivers may become irritated, impatient, and angry. They often need to be reminded that patients are not deliberately being difficult. Patients are often disruptive because they can't express their needs or wants. Careful observation may give a clue about what is causing the disruptive behavior. The patient may be comforted by simple activities, such as folding clothes or coloring. Some patients, especially women, are comforted by holding dolls or stuffed animals. The caregiver should hold the patient's hand or arm while walking. This action provides a feeling of security and prevents the patient from bolting if something frightening occurs. Busy places

often confuse and agitate patients with Alzheimer's disease or cognitive impairment, and such places as large department stores should be avoided.

<u>Environment and Medications</u>
Any unnecessary clutter should be removed from dressers, drawers, and bookshelves. Items, furniture, and rooms should be labeled if the patient is still able to read. For example, the patient's bedroom door should be labeled. If the patient is unable to read, pictures can be posted showing the use of the room or item. Dangerous items, such as knives, scissors, and matches, should be secured so that they are not accessible to the patient. If the patient is unable to climb over a gate, a child's gate can be used to block off dangerous areas.

<u>Medications</u>
In the early stages of their disease, patients may be able to manage medications if they are prepared in medication containers. However, the use of all medications should be monitored to ensure that they are used as directed. The caregiver should dispense medications if necessary. It may be necessary to disguise medications in food.

<u>Toileting</u>
Urinary and fecal incontinence usually occur over time in patients with Alzheimer's disease and cognitive impairment. However, in the early stages, certain practices, such as scheduled toileting (every 2 to 4 hours), fluid monitoring, and reducing fluid intake after dinner can help control the problem. Stool softeners may be administered to help bowel function; however, laxatives should be avoided as they may exacerbate the problem. Constipation and diarrhea can be controlled by monitoring diet. Protective coverings should be placed over the mattress and seat cushions. Disposable pads or adult diapers may eventually be necessary. The patients may resist the use of these products; different products should be tried to find one acceptable to the patient. Inappropriate

toilets such as wastebaskets should be removed if necessary. A commode may be placed in a convenient location close to a chair or the bed if necessary.

Wandering

Some patients with Alzheimer's disease or cognitive impairment tend to *wander*. This may be due to confusion. After getting lost, the patient may become frightened and hide. Patients should be registered with the Alzheimer's Association MedicAlert + Safe Return program. Patients enrolled in this program are given a MedicAlert bracelet, which they should wear at all times. It may be necessary to use alarms, latches, and locks to keep track of patients, but alarms may frighten the patient. It is best that the alarms sound in the caregiver's room rather than in the patient's room. Latches at either the top or bottom of a door are usually enough because patients usually don't think to look for a latch. In some cases, hanging a sheet or curtain over a doorway will prevent the patient from exiting through the door as patients in this condition often forget the door is there. Baby monitors may be used to keep track of the patient.

Sundowner's Syndrome

Sundowner's syndrome, also called sleep-wake cycle disruption, is a disturbance of the normal sleep-wake pattern. Some patients get up during the night and wander around the house or go through drawers or closets. They may move items around or tie them up in packages. Keeping the patient awake during the daytime can help manage the condition. In addition, turning on bright lights in the evening can help maintain the sleep-wake cycle. It may be possible to reestablish the sleep-wake cycle over one to two weeks of concerted effort. However, some people resist the process or get up at night to urinate and fail to go back to bed. Fluid restriction in the evening and/or scheduled toileting may help manage the condition. It may help to put the patient back to bed. The patient should be kept calm and relaxed at bedtime. Some patients fall asleep in a chair. In this case, a comfortable recliner placed the room may encourage the patient to sit down and fall asleep.

Pressure Ulcers

Staging

Revised regulations for the care of pressure sores in long-term care facilities were established by the Centers for Medicare & Medicaid Services (CMS) in November 2004. A standardized *staging system* was developed by the National Pressure Ulcer Advisory Panel.

- Stage I: the ulcer is an area of intact skin with red or purple discoloration. The skin may be warmer or cooler than normal. The area may be abnormally **firm** or soft in consistency. The affected area may itch or may be painful.
- Stage II: a superficial ulcer that may appear as an abrasion, blister, or slight depression. There is a partial-thickness skin loss that involves the epidermis and/or dermis.
- Stage III: a deep, full-thickness ulceration of the skin. The subcutaneous tissue may be damaged or necrotic. The ulceration may extend into the fascia, and there may be tunneling of adjacent tissue.
- Stage IV: a deep, full-thickness ulceration of the skin. The damage and necrosis of the tissue extend to muscle, bone, tendons, and joints.

Risk Factors

A list of common risk factors for pressure ulcers has been compiled by the Centers for Medicare & Medicaid Services (CMS). Many individuals have more than one risk factor. Older adults should be assessed for the following risk factors: *impairment or decreased mobility* that prevents a person from changing position; *comorbid conditions* that affect circulation or metabolism (such as renal disease, diabetes, and thyroid disease); *drugs* that interfere with healing (corticosteroids, for example); *impaired circulation* (including generalized atherosclerosis or arterial insufficiency of lower extremity); patient *refusal of care* (positioning, hygiene, nutrition, hydration, skin care); *cognitive impairment* that prevents patients from reporting *discomfort or cooperating with care*; fecal and/or urinary contamination of skin related to *incontinence*; *undernutrition, malnutrition, and/or dehydration*; presence of *healed ulcers* (healed ulcers that were stage III or IV may deteriorate and break down again).

Causes
Pressure ulcers are also called decubitus ulcers. They result primarily from pressure, but there are a number of other contributing factors:

- Pressure intensity. A capillary closing pressure of (10–32 mm Hg) is the minimum pressure needed to cause the collapse of capillaries. The collapse of capillaries contributes to the development of pressure ulcers by reducing tissue perfusion. Failure to change position while sitting or lying down can result in this pressure being exceeded.
- Duration of pressure. Low pressure for prolonged periods and high pressure for short periods can both result in pressure ulcers.
- Tissue tolerance. Tissue tolerance is the ability of the skin to tolerate and redistribute pressure. High tissue tolerance prevents anoxia. Extrinsic and intrinsic factors both have an effect on tissue tolerance. Extrinsic factors include shear, friction, and moisture. Shear is a situation in which the skin stays in place but the underlying tissue slides. Friction happens when the skin moves against bedding or other objects. Intrinsic factors include poor nutrition,

advanced age, hypotension, stress, smoking, and low body temperature.
- Shear occurs when the tissue in the deep fascia over the bony prominences stretches and slides while the overlying skin remains in place. This action damages vessels and tissue and often results in undermining. Shear is one of the most common causes of ulcers. Ulcers that result from shear are often referred to as pressure ulcers, but they are technically somewhat different. Shearing often occurs with pressure. Elevation of the head of the bed more than 30 degrees is the most common cause of shearing. The skin is held in place against the sheets while the body slides down the bed. This results in pressure and damage to the sacrococcygeal area. The blood vessels are damaged and thrombosed, leading to undermining and deep ulceration.
- Friction is a significant cause of pressure ulcers. Pressure acts in conjunction with gravity to cause shear. Friction alone causes damage only to the epidermis and dermis. This results in abrasions or denouement, which is referred to as sheet burn. Friction and pressure can act together form ulcers.

Skin Cancers

Basal cell carcinoma
Basal cell carcinoma occurs most frequently in Caucasians between the ages of 40 and 79. Most lesions develop on the face, scalp, ears, neck, arms, or hands. Lesions may recur after treatment but rarely metastasize. Lesions appear waxy at first and then ulcerate and become crusty. Treatments include electrodessication and curettage, cryosurgery, chemotherapy, laser therapy, and excision.

- 56 -

Squamous cell carcinoma

This type of lesion occurs in areas that are exposed to the sun or in areas of chronic inflammation or ulceration. The risk of metastasis is considered moderate (2–5%). At first, the lesions are indurated and erythematous, but they ulcerate and crust with time. Treatment includes excision, cryosurgery, or radiotherapy.

Malignant melanoma

There are several types of malignant melanomas: superficial, lentigo maligna, nodular, and acral lentigines. Malignant melanoma is the most serious type of skin cancer with the highest risk of morbidity and mortality. The incidence of melanoma increases with age. Melanomas often develop from moles and are irregular in shape. Melanomas are invasive and treatment involves excision. In advanced cases, palliative care is given.

Non-Cancer Skin Disorders

Herpes zoster is commonly called shingles. *Shingles* is caused by the varicella zoster virus, which remains in the nerve cells after a case of childhood chickenpox. The virus remains dormant until it is reactivated. This occurs most commonly in older adults who are immune-compromised. Initial symptoms include burning pain and redness. Painful blisters then develop along sensory nerves. The blisters often develop on a path from the spine around to the chest. However, blisters may develop on the head and face. Facial nerve involvement can result in loss of taste and hearing. Eye involvement can cause blindness. The lesions eventually crust over and heal in 2–4 weeks; however, in some cases, the affected individual may experience persistent post-herpetic neuralgia for 6–12 months. The lesions contain live virus. Contact with the virus can cause chickenpox. To prevent the development of shingles, it is recommended that individuals older than age 60 receive the herpes zoster vaccine (single dose). Treatment for shingles includes analgesia (acetaminophen), acyclovir, and Zostrix (capsaicin cream) to reduce incidence of postherpetic neuralgia.

Scabies is caused by a microscopic mite called Sarcoptes scabiei, variety hominis. The mite tunnels into the skin. This causes the development of small raised lines a few millimeters long. Although mites prefer warm areas of the body (for example, between the fingers), they can infest any area of the body. The burrowing of the mites causes intense itching. Scratching the skin can result in excoriation and secondary infections. A generalized red rash develops in some affected individuals. Scabies spreads through person-to-person contact. Staff members can spread the infection among patients. The incubation time after infection is six to eight weeks; itching usually begins in about 30 days. In most cases, only about a dozen mites are involved in an infection. However, a severe form of scabies, called Norwegian or crusted scabies, can occur in the elderly or in individuals who are immunocompromised. This type of scabies does not cause as much itching; however, the lesions can contain thousands of mites, making this type highly contagious. Treatment includes scabicides or oral medication (ivermectin) and antihistamines. Antibiotics are administered for secondary infection.

Venous dermatitis develops on the ankles and lower legs and can cause severe itching and pain. Without treatment the condition may deteriorate, resulting in the formation of ulcers. Therefore, treatment to address the symptoms is necessary. Antihistamines are administered topically to decrease itching and prevent excoriation from scratching. Low-dose topical steroids are administered reduce inflammation and itching. However, because they increase the risk of ulceration, steroids should be used only for short periods (2 weeks). Compression therapy using compression stockings is used to improve the venous return in the affected leg. Leg elevation is recommended when sitting.

Topical antibiotics (such as bacitracin) are used to reduce the danger of infection as needed. If there is a systemic infection, oral antibiotics are administered. Hypoallergenic emollients (such as petroleum jelly) improve the skin's barrier function and should be used as a preventive measure when the acute inflammation has subsided.

Contact dermatitis is a localized skin inflammation that results from contact with an allergen or irritant. The inflammation manifests as a rash that may blister and itch. The condition is commonly caused by contact with one of the following: poison oak, poison ivy, latex, benzocaine, nickel, and preservatives. However, there are many other substances and products that can cause contact dermatitis. The causative agent must be identified before treatment. A patient history must be taken to determine possible allergic reactions. A skin patch test may be performed. Corticosteroids may be administered to control inflammation and itching. Oatmeal baths may sooth the skin. Caladryl lotion is used topically to relieve itching. Antihistamines are used to reduce inflammation. Any lesions should be cleansed gently. The lesions should be evaluated for signs of secondary infection. If a secondary infection is present, antibiotics are administered. The rash should be left uncovered. The patient should be warned to avoid the allergen or irritant in the future.

Atopic dermatitis is commonly referred to as *eczema*. It is a superficial skin disorder that is chronic and inflammatory. Eczema is related to allergies and associated with xerosis, which is dry skin with impaired barrier function. It is associated with dry or cold weather, central heating (which dries the air), and the use of skin cleaners. The condition causes the skin to become red and itchy. Vesicles may develop, ooze, and crust. The skin may be rough, cracked, and scaly. Over time, the skin may darken and thicken. Lichenification, the appearance of markings from chronic scratching, may develop. To control the condition, triggers must be identified and eliminated. Treatment includes the application to weepy lesions of wet compresses soaked in aluminum acetate, lubrication of the skin three to four times each day with hypoallergenic creams, the application of topical corticosteroids for acute flare-ups, and the administration of antihistamines at night to reduce itching.

Burns

Depth of Tissue
Most burn injuries to older adults occur as a result of domestic accidents with cigarettes or stoves. About 50 percent are flame burns, 20 percent scalding injuries, 10 percent flammable liquid burns, 1 to 2 percent chemical burns, and 1 to 2 percent electrical burns. Burn injuries are often associated with impaired cognition, impaired mobility, and alcohol abuse. Burns are often deeper in older adults because the skin is thinner and healing is slower. Injuries are classified as first-, second-, and third-degree burns according to the depth of tissue affected. First-degree burns are superficial (epidermis). Second-degree burns (partial-thickness) are more serious and extend through the dermis. Third-degree burns (full-thickness) are the most severe burns and affect vasculature, muscles, and nerves.

TBSA
The American Burn Association classifies burns as minor, moderate, and major based on the percent of total body surface area (TBSA) affected. The criteria vary depending on the age of the burn victim.

- Minor burns cover less than 10 percent of the TBSA in an adult, cover less than 5 percent of the TBSA in a child or older adult, or involve a full-thickness burn that covers less than 2 percent of the body.
- Moderate burns cover 10 to 20 percent of TBSA in adults, cover 5 to 10 percent of TBSA in a child or older

adult, or involve a full-thickness burn covering 2 to 5 percent of the body.

- Major burns cover more than 20 percent of the TBSA in an adult, cover more than 10 percent of TBSA in a child or older adult, involve a full-thickness burn covering more than 5 percent of TBSA; are the result of high-voltage exposure; involve known inhalation; involve the face, eyes, ears, perineum or joints; or are associated with a significant injury.

Complications

Burn injuries, especially major burns, can affect all organs and body systems, including the cardiovascular system, urinary tract, and pulmonary system. Cardiac output may drop by 50 percent as the permeability of the capillaries increases with vasodilation and fluid leaks from the tissues. Decreased blood flow causes the kidneys to increase the production of antidiuretic hormone (ADH), which increases oliguria. Blood urea nitrogen (BUN) and creatinine levels rise. Cell destruction in the kidneys may block tubules, and hematuria may result from hemolysis. Injury to the pulmonary system may result from smoke inhalation.

Pulmonary injury is a leading cause of death from burns and is classified according to degree of damage:

- First-degree—singed eyebrows and nasal hairs with possible soot in airways and slight edema;
- Second-degree (at 24 hours)—stridor, dyspnea, and tachypnea with edema and erythema of the upper airway;
- Third-degree (at 72 hours)—worsening symptoms if the patient is not intubated. Bronchorrhea and tachypnea with edematous, secreting tissue if the patient is intubated.

Neurological: Encephalopathy may develop from lack of oxygen, decreased blood volume, and sepsis. Hallucinations, alterations in consciousness, seizures, and coma may result.

Gastrointestinal Ileus and ulcerations of the gastrointestinal mucosa often result from poor circulation. Ileus usually resolves within 48 to 72 hours, but if it returns, it is often indicative of sepsis.

Endocrine/metabolic: The sympathetic nervous system stimulates the adrenal glands to release epinephrine and norepinephrine to increase cardiac output and cortisol for wound healing. The metabolic rate increases significantly. Electrolytes, especially phosphorus, calcium, and sodium, are lost with fluid loss from exposed tissue. There is also an increase in potassium levels. An imbalance in electrolyte levels can be life threatening if the burns cover more than 20 percent of total body surface area (TBSA). Glycogen depletion occurs within 12 to 24 hours. Protein breakdown and muscle wasting occur without sufficient intake of protein.

Sensory Changes

A number of sensory changes occur in older adults. Older adults frequently experience deteriorating vision (such as presbyopia and cataracts), which prevents them from reading and navigating safely. Most people older than 60 years of age require glasses. Adults may become less sensitive to color differences (particularly blues and greens) as they age. In addition, night vision decreases. Hearing impairment may necessitate periodic cleaning of the ears or hearing aids. Taste and smell, which are both required to taste, are not usually significantly affected by normal aging. Most changes in taste and smell are caused by disease and/or drugs rather than aging. The sense of touch, including the ability to sense vibration, temperature, and pain, is usually somewhat reduced in older adults. However, it is unclear if this is a normal change or related to morbidity or drugs. A reduction in sensitivity to temperature (hot and cold) may put older adults at risk for burns, hyperthermia, and hypothermia.

Hearing Deficits

Conductive hearing deficits result from abnormalities in the structures of the outer and/or middle ear that interfere with function. Cerumen is a common cause of conductive hearing loss. *Cerumen* can result in significant hearing deficit when 95 percent occlusion occurs. Cerumen becomes hard and dry because of the atrophy of the modified apocrine glands, which thin cerumen. Removing the cerumen restores hearing. Benign growths, tympanic membrane perforation, and middle ear effusions may also impair hearing.

Sensory hearing deficits result from damage to the auditory or cochlear nerves in the inner ear. Damage may occur suddenly or progress over an extended period of time. The nerves of the ears may be damaged by Ménière's disease, viral infections, perilymph fistula, vascular occlusive disorders, and autoimmune disorders. Exposure to high-intensity sounds over an extended period of time can result in noise-induced hearing loss. *Presbycusis* is the most common hearing disorder. It is caused by physiological changes related to aging. Presbycusis causes bilateral high-frequency hearing loss.

Eye Related Problems

A cataract (opacity of the lens that interferes with vision) can occur in one eye or in both eyes. As cells die and accumulate in the eye, the lens of the eye clouds. The condition usually progresses slowly. By the age of 80, the incidence of cataracts is 50 percent. The most frequent complaint in individuals with cataracts is blurred vision without pain. Other symptoms include astigmatism, diplopia, color shift, and reduction in light transmission. A patient with cataracts should be referred to an ophthalmologist for evaluation. The condition may be surgically repaired. There are three primary types of age-related cataracts: nuclear, cortical, and posterior subcapsular. *Nuclear cataracts* are associated with myopia and tend to worsen myopia and blur vision. *Cortical cataracts* involve the anterior, posterior, or equatorial lens cortex. This condition causes vision to worsen in bright light. *Posterior subcapsular cataracts* are anterior to the posterior capsule and tend to develop in younger people or those taking corticosteroids over a long period of time. An affected eye becomes increasingly photophobic and near vision diminishes.

Glaucoma is a group of eye conditions characterized by damage to the optic nerve and vision impairment. Risk factors include being older than 40 years of age, a family history of the disease, cardiovascular disease, myopia, migraine syndromes, corticosteroid use, diabetes, and being of African American descent. Glaucoma involves an increase in intraocular pressure (normally 10–21 mm Hg) resulting from inadequate drainage of aqueous fluid. Fluid may fail to drain properly due to blockages in the drainage system and/or a decreased angle (< 45°) between the iris and cornea. There are different types of glaucoma, but the symptoms for each are similar: blurred vision, halos around lights, lack of focus, eye discomfort, headache, and difficulty seeing in low light. Referral should be made to an ophthalmologist for evaluation. Treatment may include topical beta-blockers, miotics, adrenergic agonists, carbonic anhydrase inhibitors, and prostaglandins. Surgical management includes laser trabeculoplasty, laser iridotomy, filtering procedures, trabeculectomy, and drainage implants/shunts.

Macular degeneration is the most common cause of blindness in the Caucasian population. The condition rarely occurs in other groups. There are two types of macular degeneration: dry and wet. *Dry macular degeneration* is more common and occurs when hyaline bodies, called drusen, are deposited near the retina. Dry macular degeneration begins in middle age. The condition progresses slowly and causes a loss of vision in the central part of the eye. It does not usually result in legal blindness. However, it can develop into wet macular degeneration. *Wet macular degeneration* occurs when capillaries invade the retina and grow behind the macula of the eye. Wet macular degeneration can result in legal blindness. There is no cure for macular degeneration. Vitamins A, D, and E slow the progression of dry macular degeneration. Some medications (such as Lucentis, Macugen, and Visudyne) and surgery may improve vision in individuals with wet macular degeneration. The disease appears to be heritable, and prevention is important. Eating food high in carotenoids, quitting smoking, and protecting the eyes from ultraviolet light can reduce risk.

Pain Management

There are two primary types of pain: nociceptive (acute) pain and neuropathic (chronic) pain. These two types of pain may occur together.

Nociceptive pain, also called *acute pain*, is the normal nerve response to a painful stimulus. Trauma that causes nociceptive pain can cause severe inflammation and damage to nerve endings. Nociceptive pain level is related to the type of injury and the extent of injury; the greater the injury, the greater the pain. It may be procedural pain (related to wound manipulation and dressing changes) or surgical pain (related to cutting of tissue). Nociceptive pain may be continuous or cyclic, depending upon the type of injury. Nociceptive pain is usually localized to the area of injury and resolves over time as healing takes place. This type of pain is often described as aching or throbbing. It generally responds to analgesia. If it is not controlled, over time nociceptive pain can lead to changes in the nervous system, resulting in chronic neuropathic pain.

Neuropathic pain is *chronic pain*. Neuropathic pain often results from a primary lesion in the nervous system or a dysfunction related to damaged nerve fibers. Neuropathic pain is associated with conditions such as diabetes, cancer, or traumatic injury to the nervous system. This type of pain occurs frequently in individuals with chronic wounds. The pain is often described as burning, stabbing, electric, or shooting. The pathology causing the pain is often not reversible. Pain may be visceral (diffuse or cramping pain of internal organs). Visceral pain is caused by injuries to internal organs. Neuropathic pain is often diffuse rather than localized. Neuropathic pain may also be somatic pain (involving muscles, skin, bones, and joints). Neuropathic pain is often more difficult to assess than nociceptive pain because the damage may alter normal pain responses. Neuropathic pain often responds better to antidepressants and antiseizure medications than to analgesics.

Pharmacokinetics

Pharmacokinetics involves the way in which the body affects the *absorption, distribution, metabolism, and elimination* of a drug. The process of aging affects pharmacokinetics. Absorption slows because of increased gastric pH and slower emptying time; medication may take effect more slowly and excess medication may be absorbed. The amount of intracellular and extracellular water decreases with age, resulting in a reduced distribution of water-soluble medications. Body fat increases in both men and women from early adulthood to the age of 80, so fat-soluble medications (benzodiazepines) accumulate in fat, and the half-life of drugs is prolonged. Protein-binding alterations may change half-life. Decreased cardiac output and systemic illness may affect distribution. Metabolism is affected by a decrease in liver size and a reduction in blood flow to the liver. The production of the enzymes necessary to break down medications decreases. These changes can increase the half-life of some medications by two to three times. Most drugs are eliminated through the kidneys, but renal function declines in about 65 percent of the elderly. Therefore, the half-life of most drugs is extended, necessitating lower doses.

Pharmacodynamics

Pharmacodynamics involves the effects of drugs on the body. There are a number of changes in the elderly that affect pharmacodynamics. Central nervous system changes in older adults, including changes in receptor sensitivity and in numbers of receptor sites, can result in increased adverse effects, delirium, and behavioral changes. This is especially true with benzodiazepines, opioids, alcohol, antipsychotics, anticholinergics, and barbiturates. The dosages of some drugs (such as beta-blockers) may need to be increased because a decrease in beta-adrenergic receptor function may necessitate an increased dosage of some medications. A decrease in baroreceptor function may affect the ability to increase vascular tone or cardiac output/heart rate in response to vasoactive medications, such as antihypertensives. This can result in orthostatic hypotension. Individuals on antidiabetic medications face an increased risk of hypoglycemia due to impaired glucose counter-regulation.

Drug Interactions

Drug interactions occur when one drug interferes with the activity of another in the domain of either pharmacodynamics or pharmacokinetics. In a pharmacodynamic interaction, two drugs may interact at receptor sites, causing an adverse effect or interfering with a positive effect. In a pharmacokinetic interaction, the absorption and clearance of one or both drugs are altered. This may cause delayed effects, changes in effects, or toxicity. Interactions may cause problems in a number of domains. Absorption may be increased or (more commonly) decreased. This is usually related to the effects within the gastrointestinal system. Distribution of drugs may be altered due to changes in protein binding.

Metabolism may be affected, causing changes in drug concentration. Drug interactions can impair biotransformation of the drug. Biotransformation usually occurs in the liver and gastrointestinal tract. Interactions affecting clearance may alter the body's ability to eliminate a drug, usually resulting in increased concentration of the drug.

Dosage Considerations

Gerontological dosage can be affected by a number of factors. Adverse drug effects occur two to three times more often in older adults than in younger adults. This is often related to poly-pharmacy. Since most drug trials are conducted on younger adults, information on correct dosage and drug effects in older adults is lacking. Some diseases, such as hypertension, congestive heart failure, renal failure, and diabetes, are associated with drug intolerance. In adults with these diseases, it may be necessary to use alternative medications. Drugs and nutrients may interact, impairing appetite and adversely affecting nutrition. Food and drug interactions may also alter the pharmacokinetics of nutrients or drugs, interfering with absorption, distribution, metabolism, and elimination. Mixing drugs in tube feedings or administering drugs with food increases the risk of interactions. Therefore, medications should be taken with water unless the physician instructs otherwise.

Poly-Pharmacy

The term poly-pharmacy refers to the use of multiple medications. Geriatric patients are at risk for poly-pharmacy. Patients may take the same drug under generic and brand names. They may also take drugs for one condition that are contraindicated for another condition. Patients may also take drugs that are not compatible.

There are a number of reasons for polypharmacy: Patients may receive multiple prescriptions from different doctors. Patients may also forget to tell their physician about current medications before a new prescription is issued. Patients may also use supplemental, over-the-counter, and herbal preparations in addition to prescribed medications.

Patients should be encouraged to keep a list of all current medications (prescribed and otherwise) and to take all medications to appointments. If possible, family members should be enlisted to help prevent polypharmacy in their older family members. Health-care providers must ask the patient directly about medications he or she is taking.

Oropharyngeal Dysphagia

Dysphagia is a common problem in older adults. It affects about 25 percent of hospitalized patients and 40 percent of patients in nursing homes. Dysphagia can cause anxiety about choking and can lead to malnutrition, dehydration, aspiration, and anorexia. Dysphagia is a complex problem that can be related to a number of different abnormalities. Food is masticated and then moved to the back of the throat, triggering the pharyngeal swallow reflex. At the same time, the larynx closes and the epiglottis prevents aspiration. In oropharyngeal dysphagia, this process can be impaired. Neuromuscular disorders (stroke, multiple sclerosis, and Parkinson's disease) and masses that affect the tongue, pharynx, and upper sphincter of the esophagus can cause oropharyngeal dysphagia. Affected individuals may have difficulty swallowing and may cough early in the swallow or regurgitate food into the nose. People may also exhibit dysphonia, dysarthria, and hyposalivation.

Esophageal Dysphagia

Food enters the esophagus, and peristalsis moves the food to the lower esophageal sphincter, which opens so the food can pass into the stomach. In esophageal dysphagia, people may complain of a feeling of choking and coughing late in the swallow. The swallowing process can be impaired by Parkinson's disease, achalasia, scleroderma, strictures, gastroesophageal reflux disease (GERD), and masses. Some medications (such as tetracycline, potassium, iron, nonsteroidal anti-inflammatory drugs [NSAIDs], vitamin C, alendronate, and quinidine) may also cause irritation. Diagnosis is based on history, observation, barium swallow, double-contrast upper gastrointestinal (GI) series, endoscopy, manometry (for abnormality), pH monitoring (for GERD), and videography (to assess risk of aspiration). Management includes adopting an upright position when eating; placing the food in the unaffected side of the mouth if sensory deficit is evident; taking small bites of food; adjusting food temperature (cold facilitates movement in the mouth and laryngeal swallowing, while warm facilitates other swallowing); and modifying the diet (with soft food and thickened liquids).

Nutrition

Diet Deficiencies

Diet deficiencies are common in older adults. The diets of older adults are frequently nutritionally inadequate and often contain excessive amounts of fat (especially saturated fat), cholesterol, and sodium. The diets of older adults are often deficient in protein, vitamins, and minerals. In addition, older adults are often not sufficiently hydrated. Poor diet may be related to chronic disease, lack of dentition, inability to prepare meals, or poverty. Individuals who are frail and require assistance with activities of daily living tend to have the most deficient diets, and those older than age 85 frequently have inadequate caloric intake. The diets of older adults are often deficient in calcium, vitamin D, vitamin C, vitamin B_6, thiamine, riboflavin, and all minerals, especially magnesium and zinc. Older adults may benefit from food programs (Meals on Wheels, for example) and dietary counseling. In addition, older adults should be advised to take a daily multivitamin to ensure that they receive adequate amounts of vitamins and trace minerals.

Dentition and Functional Impairment

Older patients should be assessed for dentition and functional impairment. Dentition relates directly to the ability to chew food and eat, so ill-fitting dentures, caries, or an edentulous condition may require intervention or adjustment of diet. Functional impairment may adversely affect the ability to prepare foods, eat an adequate diet, and drink an adequate amount of fluid. A functional assessment evaluates ability to participate in activities of daily living (ADLs) and instrumental activities of daily living (IADL). ADLs are those activities necessary for self-care. They include dressing, bathing, and preparing food. Inability to carry out ADLs may relate to physical impairment (paralysis, paresis, and frailty) or cognitive impairment (dementia and confusion). IADLs include such activities as managing affairs (including finances), arranging transportation, using prosthetic devices, shopping, and telephoning. The inability to carry out IADLs may relate to cognitive impairment, poverty, or inaccessibility and can prevent people from shopping for or ordering food.

Relevance to Urinary Incontinence

Dietary factors can cause urinary incontinence. Caffeine occurs naturally in coffee beans, tea leaves, and cocoa beans. Caffeine is also contained in many soft drinks, chocolate drinks, and candy. In addition, it is also an additive in many drugs (such as Excedrin, Anacin, Darvon Compound, and Fiorinal). Caffeine can increase detrusor muscle contractions, causing increased pressure that can result in urinary urgency and frequent urination. Artificial sweeteners (such as aspartame, NutraSweet, and

saccharine) are bladder irritants. Citrus foods (orange juice and cranberry juice, for example) are highly acidic and irritate the lining of the bladder. Substances that irritate the bladder can worsen overactive bladder and urge incontinence. Spicy foods, such as Mexican food, Chinese food, horseradish, and chili peppers also irritate the bladder lining. Excessive fluid intake (more than 32–48 ounces per day) can exacerbate both stress and urge incontinence. Alcohol acts directly on the bladder as a diuretic.

Dietary Management: Bowel Dysfunction

Dietary management requires identifying foods that increase bowel dysfunction. This is accomplished by having the patient make a list of the foods that he or she eats in a one-week period and keep track of bowel activity. Foods to avoid are cured or smoked meats and spicy, fatty, and greasy foods, because these often cause diarrhea and fecal incontinence. Individuals who are lactose intolerant should avoid dairy products. Caffeine, alcohol, and some artificial sweeteners (such as aspartame, NutraSweet, and saccharine) can act as laxatives, so they should be avoided. However, Splenda and stevia do not usually cause a problem. Eating several small meals instead of fewer large meals may reduce bowel contractions. Increasing fiber intake to 20 to 30 grams per day results in formed stool that is easier to control; however, too much fiber can cause bloating and gas. Therefore, fiber should be slowly added to the diet. This can be accomplished by adding whole fruits, whole grains, and vegetables to the diet. Fluid intake should be at least eight glasses per day to prevent constipation and impaction.

Constipation is usually caused by insufficient fiber in the diet. Diets high in processed foods often contain inadequate amounts of fiber. An adequate amount of fiber is 20 to 30 grams daily. There are both soluble and insoluble forms of fiber, and both add bulk to the stool. Soluble and insoluble fibers are not absorbed by the body. Some foods contain both types. Soluble fiber dissolves in liquids to form a gel-like substance. This is one reason why liquids are so important in conjunction with fiber in the diet. Soluble fiber slows the movement of stool through the gastrointestinal tract. Food sources include bananas, starches (such as potatoes and bread), cheese, dried beans, nuts, apples, oranges, and oatmeal. Insoluble fiber changes little with the digestive process and increases the speed of stool through the colon, so too much can result in diarrhea. Food sources of insoluble fiber include oat bran, seeds, skins of fruits, vegetables, and nuts.

Additional Protein and Calories

There are a number of dietary changes that can add protein to the diet. Before increasing dietary protein, comorbid conditions such as diabetes or high cholesterol should be considered; some foods, such as cheese, are high in sodium and fat, which may be restricted. Methods of increasing protein include adding meat to vegetarian dishes; adding milk powder to many foods during preparation; substituting milk for water in soups, hot cereals, and cocoa; adding cheese to dishes such as pastas and casseroles; providing high-protein drinks, such as Ensure High Protein; using peanut butter on bread and apples; and adding extra eggs to dishes such as custards and meat loaf. Methods to increase calories in the diet include using whole milk or cream rather than low-fat or nonfat milk; adding butter, sour cream, or whipping cream to foods; and eating frequent snacks.

The National Dysphagia Diet

The National Dysphagia Diet (NDD) was developed by the American Dietetic Association.

- NDD-1 (dysphagia pureed) includes foods with the consistency of pudding (such as puddings and pureed meats, fruits, and vegetables). Foods excluded from the diet include scrambled eggs, peanut butter, gelatin, yogurt with fruit, and cottage cheese. A variation of this diet is the dysphagia mixed diet. This is the NDD-1 diet with one item from NDD-2 included.
- NDD-2 (dysphagia mechanically altered) includes moist, soft, easily chewed food, such as ground or finely diced meats, tender vegetables, soft fruit, smooth moistened cereals, scrambled eggs, pancakes, and juice (thickened if needed). Excluded foods include breads, cakes, rice, peas, corn, hard fruits and vegetables, skin of fruit/vegetable, nuts, and seeds. The mechanically softened diet is a variation of the NDD-2 diet. It is the same except that it allows bread, cakes, and rice.
- NDD-3 (dysphagia advanced) includes foods with regular texture, including moist tender meats, breads, cake, rice, and shredded lettuce. Excluded are hard fruits and vegetables, corn, skins, nuts, and seeds.

Hypertension Diet

The National Institutes of Health and the National Heart, Lung, and Blood Institute have developed a program called Dietary Approaches to Stop Hypertension (DASH). Nutrient goals (based on a 2,100 calorie diet) include total fat, 27 percent of total calories; saturated fat, 6 percent; protein, 18 percent; carbohydrates, 55 percent; cholesterol, 150 mg; sodium, 1,500 to 2,300 mg; potassium, 4,700mg; calcium, 1,250 mg; magnesium, 500 mg; and fiber, 30 g. Food groups and daily servings are as follow: grains (whole grains preferred), six to eight; vegetables and fruits, four to five each; fat-free or low-fat milk/milk products, two to three; lean meat, poultry, fish six servings or less (serving = one ounce); fats and oils, two to three servings; nuts, seeds, legumes, four to five per week; and sweets and added sugars, five or less per week. Serving size depends on the food.

Diabetic Diet

Medical nutrition therapy (MNT) for diabetes includes individualized diet modifications, which may include low-fat and low-carbohydrate guidelines. Saturated fats should be restricted to less than seven percent of the total calories. Carbohydrates should be monitored through the use of carbohydrate counting or exchanges. About 45 to 65 percent of total calories should come from complex carbohydrates, and simple carbohydrates (found in sugars, pasta, potatoes, and rice) should be limited. Severely restricted carbohydrate intake (<130 mg daily) is not recommended. Sugar alcohols and nonnutritive sweeteners (such as aspartame and Splenda) are permissible. Alcohol intake should be limited to one drink per day for females and two drinks per day for males. If weight loss is an issue, women should limit intake to 1,000 to 1,200 kilocalories (kcal) per day. Men should limit their intake to 1,200 to 1,600 kcal per day. This should result in a weight loss of one to two pounds per week.

Professionalism

Confidentiality

Confidentiality is an obligation present in a professional-patient relationship. Nurses are under an obligation not to disclose information about a patient or the patient's family. Nurses must take care to safeguard information to preserve the patient's privacy. This is accomplished in a number of ways. Passwords should be required from individuals calling for information to ensure that unauthorized callers are not given information about the patient. In addition, limitations of who is allowed to visit may be set. Family members should not be apprised of the patient's condition without the patient's consent. This should not be taken for granted. Under certain conditions, it may be necessary to break confidentiality, but those circumstances are rare. The nurse must make all efforts to safeguard patient records and identification. Records on a computer should not be accessible to unauthorized personnel, and paper records must be secured.

Confidentiality Issues
Patients have a right to know that when they divulge personal information to a nurse that only those with a need to know (such as the physician and other nurses) will be provided this information. In documenting care, nurses must be sensitive to the information that they enter into the written record because many people have access to these records. The nurse is obligated to record health-related information. *Need-to-know* issues also relate to the patient's need to know about care and prognosis. Some patients may be overwhelmed by too much information, and if they are cognitively impaired, they may be confused. Older adult patients and their families should be asked how much information they want to be given. Some patients and/or their families want to know all of the details, including treatment options and expected outcomes. Others want only the basic information or don't want to discuss health issues at all.

Interviewing Skills: Pre-Interview
Prior to the interview, the nurse should review the patient's previous medical records and have a clear idea of the purpose of the interview. The nurse should outline questions to ask the patient. The patient should be interviewed alone or should be asked if he or she wants family members present. If the patient is cognitively impaired, the family may need to provide information. The nurse should obtain as much information as possible directly from the patient or from his or her observations of the patient. Family members may have to provide information, but they may overestimate or underestimate the patient's functional ability. The nurse should ensure privacy by drawing curtains, closing doors, or conducting the interview in a private setting. The nurse should sit close to the patient, face to face. The nurse should speak directly to the patient. Patients who are hearing impaired may use lip-reading to help with understanding, so the nurse should speak slowly and clearly.

Interviewing Skills: Patient
There are a number of factors that are important to a good interview. In the initial introductions, the nurse should give the patient his or her name, explain his or her role in the health-care process, and explain the purpose of the interview. The nurse should ask the patient how he or she would like to be addressed. The nurse should avoid the use of overly familiar terms such as dear. Such terms may be interpreted as condescending. The nurse should stress that the interview is confidential and explain who will have access to the information. The interview may be highly structured or flexible depending on the information required. The nurse should be able to conduct both types of interviews. The nurse should be dressed in a professional manner and wear a name tag. The nurse should assess the patient's

appearance in a nonjudgmental manner. The patient's clothing (tight or loose); cleanliness (clean or dirty); and demeanor (calm, nervous, or aggressive, for example) can indicate state of health.

Therapeutic Communication

Therapeutic communication involves face-to-face interaction that focuses on the physical and emotional health of the patient. Therapeutic communication has three purposes: 1) to gather information to assess health, 2) to assess and modify behavior, and 3) to provide health education. The nurse and patient must both be aware of the confidentiality of the communication. The nurse should not only ask questions, but observe the patient's behavior. The patient's demeanor can provide information about physical and mental health. If the patient is being evasive, he or she may look away. The nurse should ask questions to elicit information not only about the patient's health but also about the patient's attitudes and concerns. It is most important that the nurse listen empathetically to the patient. The nurse should ask "how," "who," "what," "where," and "when" questions, but "why" questions should be avoided. The nurse should ask for clarification, if needed, using reflection and rephrasing. Nontherapeutic communications should be avoided during the interview. The nurse should avoid making negative statements.

Boundary Issues

It is inappropriate for nurses to engage in sexual relations with patients. Furthermore, if the sexual behavior is coerced or the patient is cognitively impaired, it is illegal. However, more common violations with older adults include exposing a patient's body unnecessarily, using sexually demeaning gestures or language (including off-color jokes), harassment, or inappropriate touching. Nurses should take care when touching a patient. Hugging a patient in a friendly gesture can be misinterpreted.

Physical abuse is both unprofessional and illegal, but behavior can easily border on abuse without the patient being physically injured. Nurses can intimidate older adults into having procedures or treatments they don't want. Patients have the right to choose their treatment and the right to refuse treatment regardless of age. If the patient is cognitively impaired, another responsible adult (often a child or spouse) is designated to make decisions, but every effort should be made to gain the patient's cooperation. The nurse cannot make decisions for the patient against the patient's wishes or force treatment on the patient. Coercion can degenerate into physical abuse.

Nonverbal Communication

Elements of nonverbal communication include eye contact, tone, touch, gestures, and posture. Nonverbal communication can convey information from the nurse to the patient or the patient to the nurse. Eye contact maintains a sense of connection between the individuals in a conversation. The avoidance of eye contact may indicate that the person speaking is lying, uncomfortable, fearful, shy, or ashamed. The tone of voice used when speaking conveys emotion. For example, a high-pitched tone of voice may convey fear or stress. If the words spoken and tone of voice do not match, it creates unease and confusion in the listener. Touch is often reassuring, but excessive touching makes people uncomfortable and may be construed as sexual harassment. Gesture can support the meaning of spoken words. However, excessive gesturing during speech is distracting to the listener. Fidgeting with the hands and feet during an interaction can indicate nervousness. Posture can indicate emotion or lack of interest. Leaning forward during an interaction indicates interest.

Cultural Competence

Health professionals must be aware of issues related to cultural competence in dealing with patients and their families. Cultural

- 68 -

competence is the ability to interact in an effective manner with people from different cultural groups. There are four different aspects of cultural competence: 1) an individual's awareness of his or her own cultural view; 2) an individual's attitudes toward the practices of other cultural groups; 3) knowledge of the practices of other cultural groups; and 4) the ability to interact effectively with other cultural groups. Members of different cultural groups have different customs regarding eye contact, distance, and time. Some cultures avoid making eye contact, considering it rude. Individuals from these cultures may look down as a sign of respect. The space maintained between individuals varies among cultures. Members of some cultural groups stand close and some maintain a greater distance. While Americans tend to be concerned with being on time, other cultures have a more flexible view of time. It is important for health-care professionals to be sensitive to the needs of other cultural groups.

Purposes of Documentation

Documentation is written communication that provides information about the health-care patient and confirms that care was provided. Accurate, objective, and complete documentation of patient care is required by both accreditation and reimbursement agencies, including federal and state governments. Documentation serves several purposes: It carries out professional responsibility, establishes accountability, communicates information among health professionals, educates staff, provides information for research, satisfies legal and practice standards, and ensures reimbursement. While documentation focuses on progress notes, there are many other aspects to charting. Doctor's orders must be noted, medication administration must be documented on medication sheets, and vital signs must be graphed. Flow sheets must be checked off, filled out, or initialed.

The assessment carried out on admission may involve checklists or extensive documentation. Inaccurate and incomplete documentation is often an issue in malpractice cases.

Time Requirements
Documentation must be timely. Nurses should chart every one to two hours for routine care (bathing, walking), but medications and other interventions or changes in condition should be charted immediately. The failure to chart medications, especially as-needed (prn) medications, in a timely manner may result in the patient being medicated twice. This can lead to overdose. Additionally, immediate charting helps prevent nurses from forgetting to chart information or from mixing up patients. Charting in advance is illegal and can lead to unforeseen errors. Guessing that a client will have no problems and care will be routine can result in having to make corrections. The time of all interventions must be charted. Time may be a critical element, for example, in deciding if a patient should receive more pain medication or be catheterized for failure to urinate. Many health-care institutions use military time for charting. If standard time is used, the nurse should always include AM or PM with time notations.

Legibility and Clarity
Requirements for documentation include legibility and clarity. If handwritten entries are used, they must be legible and neat. Entries should be written with a blue or black permanent ink pen. Block printing should be used if handwriting is illegible. Some facilities require black ink to be used, so if unsure, nurses should use black ink. To ensure that records cannot be falsified, an erasable pen or pencil cannot be used to make entries in a patient record. To avoid falsification, a line must be drawn through empty spaces in the record. A standardized vocabulary should be used for documenting. Approved abbreviations and symbols should be used. Abbreviations and symbols can make

- 69 -

interpretation difficult and should be used sparingly.

Accuracy

A chart should always include any change in the client's condition, treatments, medications, interventions, and client responses regardless of charting format. In addition, any complaints made by the family or patient should be noted. Subjective descriptions (especially negative terms, which could be used to establish bias in court), such as tired, angry, confused, bored, rude, happy, and euphoric should not be used. The nurse should use objective descriptions, such as "Yawning two to three times a minute." If possible, clients should be quoted directly ("I shouldn't have to wait for pain medication when I need it"). If errors are made in charting (such as charting another patient's information in the record), the error cannot be erased, whited out, or otherwise made illegible. The error must be indicated by drawing a line through the text and writing "Error."

Narrative and SOAP Methods

The narrative method of documentation provides a chronological report of the patient's condition, treatment, and responses. It is an easy method of charting but may be disorganized and repetitive. In addition, if different people are making notes, they may address different issues, making it difficult to get an overall picture of the patient's progress.

SOAP stands for **s**ubjective data, **o**bjective data, **a**ssessment, and **p**lan of action. SOAP is a problem-oriented form of charting. It involves establishing goals, expected outcomes, and needs and then compiling a numbered list of problems. A SOAP note is made for each separate problem. There are four aspects to SOAP:

- subjective, the client's statement of the problem;
- objective, the nurse's observations;

- assessment, the determination of possible causes; and
- plan, the short- and long-range goals and immediate plan of care. In the case of multiple problems (edema, pain, restricted activity, and so on), this charting can be very time consuming, because each element of SOAP must be addressed. An extended version of SOAP called SOAPIER (which includes **i**ntervention, **e**valuation, and **r**evision) may be used.

PIE and Focus/DAR Methods

PIE stands for problem, intervention, and evaluation. This is a problem-oriented form of charting similar to SOAP. However, PIE is less complex than SOAP. PIE uses flow sheets in conjunction with progress notes and a list of problems. Each problem is numbered sequentially, and a PIE note is made for each problem at least one time each day or during treatment, depending on the frequency.

Focus/DAR stands for data, action, and response. This type of focused charting includes documentation about health problems, changes in condition, and concerns or events. The focus is placed on data about the injury/illness, the action taken by the nurse, and the response. Rather than following the traditional narrative linear format, the Focus/DAR format involves 3 columns (D-A-R). A DAR note is used for each focus item.

Charting: Exception and Computerized Charting

The charting by exception method was developed in response to the difficulties involved in problem-oriented charting. Charting by orientation was developed simplify charting. It includes extensive use of flow sheets. Intermittent charting is used to document unexpected findings and interventions. Because this method focuses on interventions, those problems that require no particular intervention (such as increased discomfort after ambulating) may be overlooked. Charting may not be adequate for legal challenge because lack of charting may be construed as lack of care in evaluation.

In computerized charting, all record keeping is done electronically, usually at the point of care. Computer terminals must be placed where unauthorized individuals cannot read notes being written, and access must be password protected. These systems may include clinical decision support systems (CDSS), which provide diagnosis and treatment options based on symptoms. There are some advantages to computerized charting. It is legible, tamper-proof, and tends to reduce errors as many systems signal if a treatment is missed or the wrong treatment is given.

Charting: Flow Sheets and Critical Pathways
Flow sheets are often used in combination with other methods of charting and are used to save time. They may be used to indicate completion of exercises or treatments. They usually contain areas for graphing data and may have columns or rows with information requiring checkmarks to indicate an action was completed or an observation was made.

Critical pathways are specific multidisciplinary care plans that outline interventions and outcomes of diseases, conditions, and procedures. Critical pathways are based on data and literature and best practices. The expected outcomes and sequence of interventions are delineated as well as the time line needed to achieve the outcomes. Any deviation from the pathway or expected outcomes must be documented. Critical pathways are increasingly used to comply with insurance limitations to ensure cost-effective, timely treatment.

Care Plan: Addressing Diversity
The care plan should be formatted to specifically address diversity issues. Discussions of diversity and preferences should be incorporated into the care plan during development. Studies indicate that those who are diverse in ethnicity, culture, or lifestyle are often treated differently by health-care providers in the sense that they may receive less-than-optimal care. It is the responsibility of the staff to ensure that all patients and their families receive equal quality care but with delivery of care tailored to meet the individual needs of the patients. This begins with asking staff to assess their own attitudes regarding diversity. A discussion about differences should be conducted to help people gain self-awareness and determine if their ideas are stereotypical and/or based on lack of knowledge. The original assessment by the nurse should include questions about family, country of birth, educational level, religious preferences, and native language. The nurse should explain why the questions are being asked, establishing a relationship of trust and respect that encourages the patient/family to express individual differences.

Care Plan: Patients' and Families' Rights
Patient/family rights should be incorporated into the patient's care plan. To accomplish this, the care plan needs to be designed in a collaborative effort that encourages the participation of patients and family members. There are a number of different methods that can be useful to address patients' rights. Patients and families can be included on advisory committees. Additionally, assessment tools, such as patient/family surveys, can be employed to gain insight in the issues that are important to patients and their families. Because many hospital stays are now short term, programs that include follow-up interviews and assessments are especially valuable in determining if the needs of the patient/family were addressed in the care plan.

Discharge Plan
The discharge plan should begin on admission. Older adults do not always comply with the discharge plan, so including the patient and family in the planning process

and establishing realistic goals are critical. If a patient is transferring to a long-term care facility or a home health-care program, the plan of care should be completely outlined and delivered along with copies of medical records. If a patient has had invasive procedures that increase risk for infection, the signs and symptoms of potential infection should be listed. Follow-up appointment dates with physicians, physical therapists, or other services should be included. Specific directions should be provided for all medications and treatments that are to be continued after discharge, with appropriate instruction completed prior to discharge. Contact information should be obtained from the patient so that postdischarge follow-up can be conducted, and contact information should be provided to the patient or the transfer facility.

Patient Education

Patient education is a primary concern of nursing. Written materials for older adults should be age appropriate, clearly written with a large font, and illustrated. There are commercially prepared general health materials available, but educational materials are often prepared by staff for the population served by an institution. Materials should be written and then assessed to determine if they help to meet established goals for patient understanding and compliance. All aspects of patient and family education should be documented, including the date and time of the education, the type of presentation, the handouts or material provided to the patient and/or family, and the patient's response. Older adults may be overwhelmed by packets of information and may not be able to process the information. This is especially true of adults who are weak or cognitively impaired. Therefore, the nurse should be available to review the material with the patient and demonstrate any techniques. The material should be taught in small increments, as the patient may not be able to take in too much information at one time.

Facilitation of Learning

According to the synergy model, facilitation of learning is the ability to make learning easier. Facilitation of learning requires needs assessment. In addition, the material should be structured to suit the receiver in terms of delivery and content. There are a number of levels of facilitation of learning. At level 1, the nurse is able to deliver planned educational content that is disease specific but does not have the ability to assess patient readiness to learn or abilities. The patient and his or her family are considered to be passive recipients of knowledge. At level 3, the nurse is able to individualize treatment according to the patient's and family's needs and has an understanding of different methods of teaching and learning styles. The patient's needs are considered in planning.

At level 5, the nurse has excellent understanding of teaching methods, learning styles, and assessment for learning readiness and develops an educational plan in cooperation and collaboration with others, including patients, families, and other health and allied professionals.

Team Communication

There are a number of skills that are needed to lead and facilitate communication with intra- and interdisciplinary teams. Communicating openly is essential, and all members should be encouraged to participate as valued members of a cooperative team. To facilitate the flow of information, interrupting or interpreting the point of another is discouraged. Jumping to conclusions can effectively stop communication and should be avoided. Active listening requires paying attention and asking questions for clarification. Challenging the ideas of other team members is not appropriate. It is essential to show respect for the ideas of others. Care should be taken to react and respond to facts rather than feelings. This helps prevent angry confrontations and to diffuse anger.

Clarification of information or opinions stated can help avoid misunderstandings. Unsolicited advice should not be offered, because it shows disrespect. Team members should feel comfortable about asking others for advice.

Organizational Transparency

Organizational transparency is a fairly new concept for the health-care industry, which has been historically known for concealment of data. The public has been exerting pressure to make health-care organizations more transparent as evidence about unnecessary surgery, costs, infection rates, and other negative information has been made public. The organization must be committed to transparency of pricing and quality so that both staff and patients have realistic expectations. Information that should be available includes financial information (costs and profit information), performance measures (factors that are evaluated and measured should be clearly outlined), outcomes (both positive and negative), safety records and information about safety concerns, medical records (open to individual patients), and leadership qualities and promotion (providing a clear understanding of the basis for promotion and leadership).

Patient Characteristics

According to the American Association of Critical-Care Nurses' synergy method for patient care, there are a number of patient characteristics that must be considered in matching a staff member's competencies to the requirements of the patient and the patient's family. Resiliency is the ability to recover from a devastating illness and regain a sense of stability, both physically and emotionally. Resiliency can be strengthened by faith, a positive sense of hope, and a supportive network of friends and family. Vulnerability refers to those factors that put a person at increased risk and interfere with recovery and/or compliance. These factors include anxiety, fear, lack of support, chronic illness, prejudice, and lack of information. Stability allows a patient and his or her family to maintain a state of equilibrium despite illness and challenges. Important factors contributing to stability include motivation; values; and relief from stress, conflicts, or emotional burdens. Complexity occurs when more than one system is involved. These systems can be internal (cardiac and renal systems) or external (addicted and homeless) or some combination of both (ill with poor family dynamics).

Poverty

Poverty is one of the most significant barriers to medical care, and it can affect health care in many ways. Patients may avoid routine medical visits because they don't have health insurance and don't qualify for state medical assistance. Patients may also avoid routine medical care because they are not aware that they are eligible for state medical assistance. Practitioners may not accept state medical assistance payments because of low reimbursement rates. This leaves patients with few options. Employers may not allow patients or family members of patients to take time off from work to attend medical appointments during the times that most practices are open. In many cases, people cannot afford to lose income. For these reasons, medical care may be provided by emergency departments when a crisis arises. Patients may not go for routine medical care because of lack of transportation or insufficient funds for transportation.

Hearing Impairment/Deafness

Hearing-impaired patients may have some hearing and may use hearing aids, while deaf patients typically have little or no hearing. Some hearing-impaired or deaf patients are able to lip-read, so the nurse should always face the patient and speak slowly and clearly. Gestures can be used to help convey the message but should not be used excessively. Assistive devices (such as hearing aids and writing materials) should be used to communicate with hearing-impaired patients. A normal speaking voice and short sentences should be used. Environmental noises should be kept to a minimum. If the patient is deaf, a sign language interpreter should be asked to assist. The health-care provider should face the patient, not the interpreter. A telephone device for the deaf (TDD) phone/relay service should be available for use by the patient. The health-care provider should announce his or her presence on entering a room by waving or clapping.

Visual Impairment

Visual impairment is not related to hearing, so the nurse should speak in a normal tone of voice. The nurse should face the patient so that he or she can observe the patient's facial expression. There are different degrees of visual impairment. The patient may not be able to see written materials, so different forms of materials should be available. For example, Braille handouts or large-print materials should be available. Patients with an impaired field of vision may have better vision in some areas than others, and the nurse should try to position him- or herself for the patient's advantage. The nurse should also announce his or her presence and intentions to the patient. The nurse should announce when he or she is entering or leaving the room and any actions he or she is taking. The nurse should also announce his or her position in relation to the patient and tell the patient if he or she is going to touch the patient.

Aphasia

Aphasia is the loss of ability to use and/or understand written and spoken language. It may be caused by brain tumors, brain injury, or stroke. The patient should be assessed by a speech pathologist. The symptoms depend on the area of brain damaged. There are different types of aphasia

- Global aphasia: The patient has difficulty understanding and producing language. The patient has impairments in speaking, reading, and writing, although he or she may understand gestures. The use of pictures, diagrams, and gestures to convey meaning may aid in communication. Picture charts are also helpful.
- Broca's aphasia: The patient can understand what is said but has difficulty producing language. The nurse should speak slowly, clearly, and patiently while facing the person. Picture charts may be useful to help the patient communicate.
- Wernicke's aphasia: The patient has difficulty understanding language. The patient can understand gestures and is able to produce language, although with some impairment, for example, the patient may use the wrong words. The patient may be able to write or use letter boards to assist communication.

Dysarthria

Dysarthria is unclear speech caused by slurring. In older adults, dysarthria may be related to missing teeth; neurological disorders (such as Parkinson's, Huntington's, and multiple sclerosis); stroke; Bell's palsy; alcohol intoxication; brain injury; or excessive drug intake (such as narcotics and phenytoin). Dysarthria is not related to intelligence level or hearing ability, so the nurse should use age-appropriate vocabulary and materials and speak in a normal tone of voice. When conversing, the nurse should face the patient so that he or she can observe the patient's gestures and facial expressions. This practice will facilitate communication. Some patients with dysarthria use materials to aid communication (flip charts, letter boards, computer programs, or speech-generating devices). If this is the case, these materials should be available and the nurse should be knowledgeable about their use. If the patient is unable to speak, perhaps due to oral surgery or tracheotomy, then the nurse should determine if the patient is able to indicate yes/no by blinking or nodding. In general, questions requiring a yes/no answer are easiest for patients with dysarthria. It's important not to hurry the patient.

Role of Interpreters

Interpreters play an important role in improving medical care for patients who do not speak English. The patient's access to care and compliance to treatment can be compromised if he or she does not speak English or speaks English poorly. If the patient population of a health-care center draws from a minority population, the center should take steps to improve communication between staff and patients. For example, the center could hire bilingual staff; provide language classes for existing staff; and provide translated materials (treatment guidelines, pamphlets, and symbol-based signs, for example). Many practices depend on the patient's family members to translate. However, this is often not a good solution. Children often lack the maturity to assume this responsibility, and family members may not have the interest. Also, the family members may not have an adequate vocabulary or understanding to translate effectively. This could lead to serious misunderstandings. Interpreters should have training in medical vocabulary. Translation resources can be pooled among a number of practices/institutions to control costs.

Essential Duties of Nurses
The American Nurses Association's Scope and Standards of Gerontological Nursing Practice includes many skills, such as providing care, managing care, advocating for the patient, and researching ways to improve care. Education is an essential role of the gerontological nurse. Duties outlined by the Scope and Standards of Gerontological Nursing Practice include utilizing data,

information, and knowledge to develop a patient care plan; assessing information for diagnosis; influencing health outcomes; planning care to provide appropriate treatment; implementing interventions and evaluating treatment progress; evaluating the quality of care; self-assessment of abilities and performance in relation to professional standards; keeping up to date in the field; providing care in an ethical manner; working collaboratively with patients, family, caregivers, and interdisciplinary team members; utilizing research to provide evidence-based care; and providing and promoting safe and cost-effective care to all patients.

Standards of Advance Practice
The gerontological nurse must adhere to the standards of advance practice. These standards provide the guidelines for practice and describe the responsibilities of the gerontological nurse. The standards outline the values and priorities of the profession.

- In the care process, the nurse assesses, develops, and implements a plan of care and evaluates the patient's response; the nurse must use the scientific method and national standards as the basis for care.
- In establishing priorities, the nurse provides education and encourages the patient and his or her family to take an active role in self-care. The nurse must be sure that the patient is able to make informed decisions. The nurse must assist the patient through all aspects of health care to ensure patient safety and optimal care.
- Collaboration is essential. As a member of an interdisciplinary health team, the nurse must consult with other team members when appropriate.
- Documentation: The nurse must keep accurate, legal, and legible records. The nurse must ensure that patient confidentiality is maintained. The nurse must not provide medical

records to other parties unless the patient first signs a release form.

- Patient advocacy: The nurse should advocate not only for individual patients under his or her care, but also for patients at the state and national level. The nurse should strive to facilitate patient access to care and improve the quality of care.
- Continuous quality improvement: The nurse must take part in continuing education and continuous evaluation and quality review.
- Research and education: The nurse must initiate and participate in research and use the results of research in clinical practice.

Thermoregulation is the ability of an organism to maintain an optimum temperature in the presence of a variety of external conditions. The body maintains its core temperature by balancing heat gains and losses. The feedback system of the human body regulates the temperature so that it remains at a nearly constant 98.6 degrees Fahrenheit (F). Thermoregulation is controlled by the central nervous system. Generally, thermoregulation is possible when the environmental temperature is between 68 degrees F and 130 degrees F. When thermoregulation breaks down and body temperature increases significantly above normal, hyperthermia occurs. When the temperature drops significantly below normal, hypothermia occurs. Older adults do not thermoregulate as efficiently as younger individuals. Older adults are less tolerant of changes in ambient temperature. Older adults should be kept warm and comfortable during physical examinations.

Skin care
The skin of older adults is often friable and bruises easily. Therefore, it should be treated with care. Excessive palpitation and pulling should be avoided. The skin should be examined for lesions or indications of pressure ulcers. Older adults often have benign skins lesions, including, acrochordons (skin tags), actinic keratoses, cherry hemangiomas, dermatofibromas, lentigines (liver spots), nevi (moles), sebaceous hyperplasia, and seborrheic keratoses. Some of these types of lesions, such as actinic keratoses, are precancerous and should be examined carefully as they may become squamous cell or basal cell carcinoma. Malignant melanoma can occur in individuals of any age. These lesions occur most frequently on the torso, head, and neck of males and the legs of females.

Positioning
Many adults have mobility problems, a limited range of motion, and difficulty maintaining certain positions. Physical limitations differ for different patients. Each patient should be positioned in the most comfortable position. Changes of position should be minimized.

Sensory impairment
Sensory impairments include deficits in vision, hearing, and sense of touch. These problems should be assessed early. If deficits are known, accommodations should be made. If the patient wears a hearing aid, the nurse should request that the patient wear it during the exam. The room should be quiet and free of distraction.

Extremities
Extremities should be examined using modified movements. Force must not be used. For example, care should be taken when pushing a limb into flexion or extension. The nurse should not ask the patient to do things that put too much stress on the limbs. For example, the patient should not be asked to do deep bends. Older patients may have decreased range of motion, slower reflexes, and poor balance. The nurse should always ensure that the limbs are supported during inspection.

Physical Assessment Guidelines

Older patients may have a decreased respiratory force and cough reflex and may be short of breath. Chest inspection may have to be modified as a consequence. Inspection may take longer in order to allow the patient to rest between deep breaths.

Abdominal inspection should be done with care. Older adults may have a decreased sensation of pain on deep palpation. There is less cushioning for the liver, so the area should be palpitated gently to prevent damage to the tissue.

Genitalia should be examined, but older adults may be embarrassed, so the nurse should explain the need for the procedure. Older women often have vaginal atrophy with decreased lubrication, so a smaller speculum should be used, and it should be well lubricated. Perianal pruritis is common in older adults, but they are often embarrassed to talk about it. The nurse should ask if there is any itching in the area.

Auscultation

This procedure involves the use of a stethoscope to listen to the movement of air or fluid within the body. The sounds are characterized according to intensity (loudness), frequency (pitch), and quality. Auscultation is commonly used to assess the functioning of the heart and lungs. It is also used to determine if circulatory impairment (bruit) is present and to listen to bowel sounds.

Palpation

Palpation involves using the fingertips to evaluate the characteristics of a particular part of the body. Hardness, temperature, swelling, size, and mobility can be assessed by palpation. Care should be taken when palpating the area over the liver; excessive pressure should be avoided. In some cases, sound may be felt as vibrations.

Percussion

Percussion is a technique in which the fingers of one hand are laid flat against the skin and tapped with the finger tips of the other hand. This causes sound to resonate. Percussion is most commonly used to assess organ size or changes in tissue density. Care should be used over the liver, spine, and bladder.

Problem-Based Psychosocial Assessment

Older adults often present with myriad health problems. If this is the case, it can be effective to use a problem-based psychosocial assessment that focuses on finding solutions for particular problems. It is necessary to take a thorough patient history. When appropriate, family members and caregivers should be consulted to aid in the development of a problem list. A complete exam is still conducted because it might identify problems that the patient is unaware of or has neglected to mention. However, the focus remains on the problem list generated. Items should be ranked according to their severity. This ensures that the most serious issues are assessed before less serious issues. Once a problem is identified, then differential diagnoses are developed. A particular problem may be due to physical and/or psychosocial elements. For example, urinary problems may relate to dehydration, lack of mobility, poor hygiene, medications, disease, or a combination of these factors. Appropriate diagnostic tests, further assessments, and interventions are completed as needed to diagnose and resolve the problems.

Sexually Transmitted Diseases

Older adults are more active and healthier than ever before, and the incidence of sexually transmitted diseases among older adults is increasing. However, older adults often practice unsafe sex and fail to use condoms. The Centers for Disease Control has developed six steps to prevent and control the spread of sexually transmitted diseases:

- Step 1: identify symptomatic and asymptomatic infected persons;
- Step 2: diagnose and treat all infected individuals;
- Step 3: prevent the infected individual from infecting sex partners through evaluation, treatment, and counseling;
- Step 4: provide preexposure vaccination to individuals at risk;
- Step 5: educate individuals at risk about ways to prevent infection; and
- Step 6: obtain sexual histories of patients and assess their risk. The 4-P approach (omitting pregnancy) to questioning is advocated: **p**artners, gender and number; **p**rotection, methods used; **p**ractices, type of sexual practices (oral, anal, vaginal) and use of condoms; and **p**ast history of sexually transmitted diseases.

Asthma

Asthma in seniors may be a continuing condition from childhood, but it may also develop in older people. Asthma may be diagnosed as a new disorder in seniors. The symptoms of asthma include wheezing, tightness of the chest, shortness of breath, and coughing. The symptoms are episodic and do not appear continually through the day. The symptoms usually worsen at night and while exercising. Airborne allergens can exacerbate or trigger the symptoms. The patient may exhibit allergic rhinitis and/or atopic dermatitis. Physical examination may show hyperextension of the patient's thorax. The condition tends to be hereditary; the patient may have relatives with the disorder. The symptoms of asthma are not always present. A diagnosis of asthma cannot be excluded because symptoms are absent at the time of examination. Episodic airflow obstruction that is partly reversible is diagnosed by spirometry. Further tests include pulmonary function studies, bronchoprovocation, allergy tests, and chest x-rays. In seniors, asthma is often complicated by age and cormorbid conditions.

Hypertension

The risk of developing hypertension begins to increase in middle age. The risk increases with increasing age. Hypertension has long-term health risks. Individuals with hypertension have a higher risk of heart disease, stroke, peripheral vascular disease, and kidney disease. Physicians have been encouraged to treat hypertension aggressively. Lifestyle changes may be recommended in order to lower hypertension. Lifestyle changes include exercise, losing weight, eating a healthy diet (by reducing salt and fat intake), and quitting smoking. Drug therapy is usually required for hypertension. The choice of medication depends on the patient's age, severity of the condition, and comorbid conditions. There are a number of classes of drugs used to treat hypertension, including diuretics, beta-blockers, calcium antagonists, angiotensin-converting enzyme (ACE) inhibitors, angiotensin receptor blockers, and alpha-1 adrenergic antagonists. Individuals with hypertension may be reluctant to take medication because they feel no symptoms. It is up to the health-care provider to explain why taking medication is essential.

Braden Scale

Pressure Sore Risk
The Braden scale is used to assess a patient's risk of developing pressure sores. The scale has been clinically validated and is widely used. The scale rates six different areas on a scale of 1 to 4. The sub-scores from all areas are added together to create a total score. The patient's risk of developing pressure sores is determined by the total score. The best (and highest) score is 23. Lower ratings indicate a higher risk of developing pressure sores. If the patient has a score of 16 or lower, prevention protocols should be initiated. The worst score obtainable is 6: This patient has a

very strong possibility of developing pressure sores.

Sensory Perception, Moisture, and Mobility

The first four assessment areas of the Braden scale are sensory perception, moisture, activity, and mobility. Patients are rated on a scale of 1 to 4:

- Sensory perception.
  - Completely limited (unresponsive to pain or has limited ability to feel)
  - Very limited (responds to painful stimuli and moans)
  - Slightly limited (responds to verbal commands but has limited communication) 4. No impairment
- Moisture
  - Moist constantly
  - Very moist (linen change required each shift)
  - Occasionally moist (linen change required each day)
  - Rarely moist

Activity

- Bed bound
- Chair bound
- Walks occasionally (short distances)
- Walks frequently

Mobility

- Completely immobile
- Very limited (makes occasional slight position changes)
- Slightly limited (makes frequent slight position changes)
- No limitations

Nutrition Pattern and Friction and Shear

The last two areas assessed by the Braden scale are usual nutrition pattern and friction and shear. Patients are rated on a scale of 1 to 4:

- Usual nutrition pattern
  - Very poor (eats less than half of meals, inadequate protein intake, and inadequate hydration)
  - Inadequate (eats about half of food with three protein serving or not enough liquid or tube feeding)
  - Adequate (eats less than half of meals and four protein servings)
  - Excellent
- Friction and shear (three parameters only)
  - Problem moving (skin frequently slides down the sheets, needs help to move)
  - Potential problem (moves weakly or needs some assistance, skin slides somewhat during moves)
  - No apparent problem

Physical/Psychosocial Assessment

Patients with signs or symptoms of dementia or short-term memory loss should have a cognitive assessment. The Mini-Mental State Exam (MMSE) or the Mini-Cog test is commonly used for this purpose. Both tests require the patient to carry out specified tasks.

Mini-Mental State Exam (MMSE): The tasks for this test include remembering and later repeating the names of three common objects; counting backward from 100 by 7s; spelling the word "world" backward; naming items as the examiner points to them; providing the location of the examiner's office, including city, state, and street address; repeating common phrases; copying a picture of interlocking shapes; and following simple three-part instructions (for example, picking up a piece of paper, folding it in half, and placing it on the floor).

Mini-Cog: The tasks for the Mini-Cog test are as follows: remembering and later repeating the names of three common objects and drawing the face of a clock with all 12 numbers with the hands indicating a time specified by the examiner.

The 1 To 10 Pain Scale

Pain is subjective. Pain threshold (the smallest stimulus that produces the sensation of pain) and pain tolerance (the maximum amount of pain that a person can tolerate) vary among individuals. The most commonly used pain assessment tool is the 1 to 10 pain scale (0 = no pain, 1–2 = mild pain, 3–5 = moderate pain, 6–7 = severe pain, 8–9 = very severe pain, and 10 = excruciating pain). However, there are other aspects to pain assessment. Assessment includes collecting information regarding onset, duration, and intensity. Identifying those things that trigger pain and those things that relieve pain can be very useful when developing a plan for pain management. Individual reaction to pain differs. Some patients may cry and moan with minor pain, and others may exhibit little difference in behavior when truly suffering; thus, judging pain by the behavior of the patient can lead to the wrong conclusions.

Rating Pain in the Cognitive Impaired

Patients with cognitive impairment may not be able to verbalize pain. The patient may not even be able to indicate the degree of pain by using a face scale with pictures of smiling to crying faces. The Pain Assessment in Advanced Dementia (PAINAD) scale may be helpful. Nonverbal behavior can indicate pain and degree of pain. The patient should be carefully observed for the following signs:
- Respirations: Patients often have more rapid and labored breathing as pain increases. The patient may have short periods of hyperventilation or Cheyne-Stokes respirations.
- Vocalization: Patients in pain may speak quietly and reluctantly. They may moan or groan. As pain increases, patients may call out, moan or groan loudly, or cry.
- Facial expression: Patients may appear sad or frightened or may frown or grimace, especially during activities that increase pain.

- Body language: Patients may be tense and may fidget or pace. As pain increases, patients may become rigid, clench their fists, or lie in a fetal position. They may become increasingly combative.
- Consolability: Patients are less distractible or less consolable as pain increases.

Assessing Falls

The American Geriatrics Society Guidelines for the Prevention of Falls in Older Persons has established a protocol for dealing with older patients. All geriatric patients should be asked if they have had falls in the past year. If no falls have occurred, no intervention is needed. If one fall has occurred, the patient should be assessed for gait and balance. The nurse should administer the get-up-and-go test, in which the patient stands up from a chair without using his or her arms for assistance, walks across the room, and returns. If the patient is steady, no further assessment is needed. If the patient demonstrates unsteadiness, further assessment to determine the cause is necessary. If the patient has had multiple falls, a full assessment should be completed, including history, vision, neurological status, muscle strength, joint function, mental status, reflexes, cardiovascular status (including rate and rhythm), postural pulse, and blood pressure. Referral to a geriatric specialist may be appropriate.

Nutrition Assessment

The MNA (Mini-Nutritional Assessment) by Nestlé Nutrition is designed for nutritional assessment of adults older than age 65. The MNA is only valid for that population. It is a screening and assessment tool to determine the risk for malnutrition. It is composed of 15 questions about dietary habits and four measurements, including body mass index (BMI) using height and weight and midarm and calf circumference.

The Nutritional Screening Initiative is another tool used to assess nutrition in geriatric patients. It screens for dietary information as well as social and environmental factors, such as whether the person eats alone, prepares meals, drinks alcohol, and has sufficient income.

The Subjective Global Assessment tests nutritional status by a thorough history and physical examination. The history assesses weight change, dietary intake, gastrointestinal symptoms, and functional impairment. The results of this assessment tool are evaluated subjectively, and scores are assigned to determine the extent of malnutrition risk.

Risk for Pressure Sores

The Norton scale assesses risk for pressure ulcers based on scores in five categories. Each category is rated on a scale from 1 to 4. The scores for all categories are added together. A higher number indicates higher risk. A score of 14 or greater indicates that the patient is at high risk. The scale is used for periodic assessment (on a daily or weekly basis) so that patients at risk can be identified quickly and interventions instituted.

Norton Scale

Condition	1	2	3	4
Physical	Good	Fair	Poor	Very poor
Mental	Alert/responsive	Apathetic	Confused	Stuporous
Activity	Ambulatory	Walks with help	Nonambulatory/chair bound	Bedridden
Mobility	Full mobility	Slightly limited	Very limited	Immobile
Incontinence	None	Occasionally	Urinary incontinence	Fecal and urinary incontinence

The Barthel Index of Activities of Daily Living

The Barthel index of activities of daily living is a tool used to assess the functional ability of older adults. It is used to assess the person's disabilities and need for assistance. There are 10 categories that are rated on a scale of 0 to 15 (100-point scale) or 0 to 3 (20-point scale) with lower scores indicating greater levels of dependence. Higher scores indicate greater levels of independence. This scale is sometimes modified by institutions, so it may vary somewhat. The 10 categories usually include the following:
- Feeding (includes need to cut food)
- Mobility
- Personal grooming
- Toileting (getting on and off toilet, wiping, and managing clothes)
- Urinary control
- Fecal control
- Ascending and descending stairs
- Ambulatory status on level ground (or if wheelchair bound, the ability to propel the wheelchair)
- Transferring, sitting up in bed
- Bathing

IADLs

Instrumental activities of daily living (IADLs) describe an assessment tool used to measure the ability to perform eight activities necessary for an adult to function independently. This tool helps to determine the need for supportive services. Scores are assigned as 0 (cannot do independently) or 1 (minimal or adequate degree of ability), so the total score ranges from 0 to 8. A higher score indicates greater independence. Abilities that are measured include the following:
- Telephone use (ability to look up and/or call numbers)
- Shopping for food, clothes, or needed items
- Food preparation (ability to plan diet and prepare food)
- Housekeeping (ability to perform all or some household duties)
- Laundry (ability to wash all or some personal laundry)
- Transportation availability (ability to drive or use public transportation)
- Medication (ability to manage prescriptions and take medications)
- Financial responsibility (ability to keep track of finances, pay bills, and budget).

Katz Index and the Palliative Performance Scale

The Index of Independence of Activities of Daily Living (Katz Index) assesses the patient's abilities to perform certain activities, but does not use scores. The patient is evaluated in six areas (bathing, dressing, toileting, transfer, continence, and feeding). The index is used to assess the person's need for assistance and the progression of the disease and/or disability.

The Palliative Performance Scale assesses the functional ability of older adults receiving palliative care. Categories are assessed by percentage of ability ranging from 0 percent (death) to 100 percent. Lower percentages indicate functional impairment. The scores are used as a guide to determine probable life expectancy with 60 to 100 percent at 108 days, 30 to 50 percent at 41 days, and 10 to 20 percent at 6 days; survival rates have been primarily correlated with cancer rather than other terminal illness. Categories include ability to ambulate, activity level and evidence of disease, self-care, intake, and level of consciousness.

Confusion Assessment Method

The Confusion Assessment Method is used to assess the development of delirium and is intended for use by those without psychiatric training. The tool covers nine factors. Some factors have a range of possibilities, and others are rated only as to whether the characteristic is present, not present, uncertain, or not applicable. The tool provides room to describe abnormal behavior. Factors assessed include onset, attention, thinking, level of consciousness, orientation, memory, perceptual disturbances, psychomotor abnormalities, and the sleep-wake cycle. Delirium is indicated if there is an acute onset with fluctuating attention, disorganized thinking, or altered consciousness.

- Onset: Acute change in mental status
- Attention: Inattentive, stable, or fluctuating
- Thinking: Disorganized, rambling conversation, switching topics, illogical
- Level of consciousness: Altered, ranging from alert to coma
- Orientation: Disoriented (person, place, time)
- Memory: Impaired
- Perceptual disturbances: Hallucinations, illusions
- Psychomotor abnormalities: Agitation (tapping, picking, moving) or retardation (staring, not moving)
- Sleep-wake cycle: Awake at night and sleepy in the daytime.

Digit Repetition Test and The Time and Change Test

The digit repetition test is used to assess the ability to pay attention. The patient is asked to listen to numbers and then repeat them. The nurse starts with two random single-digit numbers. If the patient gets this sequence correct, the nurse then states three numbers and continues to add one number each time until the patient is unable to repeat the numbers correctly. People with normal intelligence can usually repeat five to seven numbers, so scores of less than five indicate impaired attention.

The time and change test assesses dementia in older adults. The test is effective in diverse populations. Patients are shown a clock face set at 11:10 and have one minute to make two attempts at stating the correct time. The patient is then given change (seven dimes, seven nickels, and three quarters) and asked to give the nurse $1.00 from the coins. The patient has two minutes and two tries to make the correct change. Failing either or both tests is indicative of dementia.

The Trail Making Test

The trail making test (parts A and B) assesses brain function and indicates increasing dementia. It is useful for detecting early Alzheimer's disease. Individuals who do poorly on part B often need assistance with activities of daily living. In part A, circles containing the numbers 1 through 25 are scattered across the page. The numbers are not in sequence. The patient is asked to draw a continuous line to connect (in ascending order) the circles (starting with 1 and ending with 25). Part B is slightly more complex. The numbers 1 through 12 and letters A through L are contained in circles. These circles are scattered about the page. The patient is asked to draw a continuous line alternating between numbers and letters in ascending order (1-A-2-B . . .). Both parts of the test are scored according to the number of seconds required for completion. In part A, a score of 29 seconds is average, and a score of greater than 78 indicates deficiency. In part B, a score of 75 seconds is average, and a score of greater than 273 seconds indicates deficiency.

GDS

The Geriatric Depression Scale (GDS) is a self-assessment tool designed to identify older adults with depression. The original test is now in the public domain. The test can be used to assess individuals with normal cognition and individuals with mild to moderate impairment. The test poses 15 questions to which patients answer yes or no. A score with more than five yes answers is indicative of depression. The questions are as follows:

- Are you basically satisfied with your life?
- Have you dropped many of your activities and interests?
- Do you feel your life is empty?
- Do you often get bored?
- Are you in good spirits most of the time?
- Are you afraid that something bad is going to happen to you?
- Do you feel happy most of the time?
- Do you often feel helpless?
- Do you prefer to stay at home rather than going out and doing new things?
- Do you feel you have more problems with memory than most people?
- Do you think it is wonderful to be alive now?
- Do you feel pretty worthless the way you are now?
- Do you feel full of energy?
- Do you feel that your situation is hopeless?
- Do you think that most people are better off than you are?

Bladder Diary

A bladder diary is a complete daily record of all urinations and all episodes of urinary incontinence. The diary is usually kept for 3 to 5 days as part of the urological assessment. The diary contains the time of urination, the amount of urination, fluid intake, and incontinence. The time is recorded to determine *patterns of urination*. The amount of urine passed should be estimated (small, medium, or large). Fluid intake should be recorded in order to determine if fluids are contributing to incontinence or urinary problems. Incontinence should be characterized by estimations of amount. A small volume of less than 30 ml is enough to wet underwear. A moderate volume of 30 to 60 ml is enough to soak underwear with overflow down legs. A large volume of more than 60 ml is usually enough to soak clothes and run onto the floor or furniture. Incontinence should be characterized by activity and strength of urge to help determine the type of incontinence.

Bowel Diary

A bowel diary is a complete daily record of all defecations and episodes of fecal incontinence or flatus. The diary is usually kept for three to five days as part of the intestinal assessment and includes the time of each bowel movement; the type of bowel movement (hard lumps, sausage-shaped, cracked sausage-shaped, smooth and snakelike, soft blobs, fluffy pieces, or liquid); the amount of stool; abnormalities (such as blood or mucus and the need for finger splinting or straining); fecal incontinence (characterized by amount and type and activity at the time of incontinence); flatal incontinence; intake of both food and fluids (to determine if intake relates to bowel activities); and medications (including laxatives, vitamins, and any over-the-counter preparations).

AIMS

The Abnormal Involuntary Movement Scale (AIMS) is a tool used to evaluate patients for tardive dyskinesia. Tardive dyskinesia is a movement disorder caused by some antipsychotic medications. Before or after the formal examination, the patient is observed at rest (as in the waiting area) for comparison. The examination procedure includes having the patient perform a number of activities, such as sitting in specific positions, opening his or her mouth, sticking out his or her tongue, standing, and walking while the nurse rates a number of movements on a scale of 0 (none) to 4 (severe). The severity of facial and oral movements, extremity movements, and trunk movements is rated. A score of 2 or higher in two or more movements or a score greater than 3 in one movement is positive for tardive dyskinesia. The overall severity is then assessed (based on the above scores), including patient's degree of incapacitation and patient's awareness of abnormal movements. The last part of the exam asks about dental status.

Cholesterol Levels

Cholesterol is a naturally occurring substance. Cholesterol is necessary for the development of healthy cell membranes and the production of hormones. However, if too much cholesterol is present, it can adhere to the arteries and clog the vessels. This process is the start of heart disease. Cholesterol level is determined by blood test. Three measurements are generated from cholesterol testing: total cholesterol, high-density lipoproteins (called HDLs), and low-density lipoproteins (called LDLs). HDLs are referred to as good cholesterol. This type of cholesterol prevents cholesterol from adhering to the arteries. LDLs are referred to as bad cholesterol. This type of cholesterol adheres to the artery walls. A total cholesterol score of less than 150 is optimum. A total cholesterol score of 240 or higher is in the high-risk category. An HDL of 45 or less is also in the high-risk category. Cholesterol increases with age. High alcohol intake, a sedentary lifestyle, cigarette smoking, and a high-fat diet can increase cholesterol level. Certain diseases (such as hypothyroidism, chronic kidney failure, and diabetes) are also associated with elevated LDL cholesterol.

Colorectal Cancer

Colorectal cancer is also called colon cancer and large bowel cancer. Growths may occur in the colon, rectum, or appendix. Cancer growths are thought to develop from adenomatous polyps. Symptoms include a change in bowel function (constipation or diarrhea), a change in stool shape, a feeling of incomplete bowel movement, the presence of bright red blood in the feces, and the presence of mucus in the feces. If the bowel is obstructed, the patient may experience abdominal pain and distention and vomiting. Diagnosis is usually made by colonoscopy. Treatment usually involves surgery and chemotherapy. Risk factors include a family history of the disease, a genetic predisposition, a history of polyps, and a history of inflammatory bowel disease. Screening tests includes fecal occult blood test (yearly), flexible sigmoidoscopy (every five years), colonoscopy performed (every 10 years), and double-contrast barium enema (every five years).

Glucose and Hemoglobin A1c

Glucose is manufactured by the liver from ingested carbohydrates and is stored as glycogen for use by the cells. If glucose intake is inadequate, glucose can be produced by the breakdown of muscle and fat tissue. This can lead to increased wasting. High levels of glucose are indicative of diabetes mellitus. Fasting blood glucose levels are used to diagnose and monitor glucose levels:

- Normal values: 70–99 mg/dL
- Impaired: 100–125 mg/dL
- Diabetes: >126 mg/dL

A number of different conditions are associated with increased glucose levels: stress, renal failure, Cushing's syndrome, hyperthyroidism, and pancreatic disorders. Some medications (such as steroids, estrogens, lithium, phenytoin, diuretics, and tricyclic antidepressants) may increase glucose levels. Other conditions (adrenal insufficiency, liver disease, hypothyroidism, and starvation, for example) can decrease glucose levels.

Hemoglobin A1c is composed of hemoglobin A plus a glucose molecule. Hemoglobin holds on to excess blood glucose, so hemoglobin A1c level is used primarily to monitor long-term diabetic therapy. The normal value is less than six percent and a value of greater than seven percent is elevated.

Urinalysis

Color: Urine is usually pale yellow/amber. Urine darkens when it is concentrated or when other substances are present.

- Appearance: Urine is usually clear but may be slightly cloudy.
- Odor: The odor should be slight. Bacteria may impart a foul smell.
- Specific gravity: The specific gravity of urine is between 1.015 and 1.025

but may increase if protein levels increase or if there is fever, vomiting, or dehydration.

- pH: The pH of urine usually ranges from 4.5 to 8 (average 5–6).
- Sediment: Urine may contain red cell casts from acute infections, broad casts from kidney disorders, and white cell casts from pyelonephritis. Leukocytes at a concentration of greater than 10 per ml^3 are present in the case of urinary tract infection.
- Glucose, ketones, protein, blood, bilirubin, and nitrates: These values should all be negative. Urine glucose may increase with infection. Frank blood may be caused by some parasites and diseases but also by some drugs, smoking, excessive exercise, and menstrual fluids. Increased red blood cells may result from lower urinary tract infections.
- Urobilinogen: Values of urobilinogen range from 0.1 to 1.0 units.

Pain Management

The type of pain determines the methods used to manage it. Acute pain occurs as a biological response to illness or injury and usually responds to opiates. Chronic pain is defined as pain that lasts three months or more or one month longer than usual for a particular condition. Chronic pain cannot usually be completely relieved. However, the patient can use methods to manage chronic pain. Pain may be dull, sharp, cramping, shooting, burning, constant, or recurrent. The three primary types of chronic pain include nociceptive (usually responds well to central-acting analgesia), neuropathic (often responds poorly to analgesia), and psychogenic (may be difficult to treat because of patient resistance). Identifying the type of pain and triggers or aggravating conditions is important to help the patient avoid inducing pain. Pain management programs depend on the type of pain and may include diet and exercise; psychological counseling;

acupuncture; analgesia (nonsteroidal anti-inflammatory drugs [NSAIDs], opiates, corticosteroids, and acetaminophen); antidepressants (amitriptyline); and anticonvulsants (carbamazepine and valproic acid).

World Health Organization Pain Ladder

The World Health Organization (WHO) Pain Ladder has been established as guidance for pain management. Medications are usually given every three to four hours around the clock to prevent breakthrough pain.

Level 1—Mild pain
Pain management usually begins with acetaminophen or aspirin followed by NSAIDs. Adjuvant drugs may be administered. There are a number of different NSAIDs. There are individual differences in the response to drugs, so patients should be monitored carefully and medication changed if indicated.

Level 2—Mild to moderate pain
Aspirin or acetaminophen is given with codeine and adjuvant medication. Medications include hydrocodone, oxycodone, and tramadol.

Level 3—Moderate to severe pain
Opioid drugs (morphine, fentanyl, and oxycodone) are given to control moderate to severe pain. Some nonopioid drugs and adjuvant drugs may also be used. Adjuvant drugs include NSAIDs, anticholinergics, anticonvulsants, antiemetics, antipruritics, and corticosteroids.

Diabetes: Renal Complications

The American Diabetes Association Clinical Practice Recommendations for preventing renal complications of diabetes are as follows:

Screening and diagnosis:
All individuals who have had type 1 diabetes for five or more years and all individuals with type 2 diabetes should have an annual urine albumin test. Serum creatinine should be assessed annually to estimate glomerular filtration rate (GFR) and determine degree of chronic kidney disease.

Treatment:
Treatment includes angiotensin-converting enzyme (ACE) inhibitors or angiotensin receptor blockers (ARBs) (with monitoring of serum creatinine and potassium) and reduction of protein intake to 0.8 to 1.0 g/kg/body weight per day in the early stages of chronic kidney disease and 0.8 g/kg/body weight per day in cases of advanced chronic kidney disease.

Glucose monitoring:
Maintaining normal steady glucose levels is critical to avoid renal disease. Twenty to forty percent of patients with persistent albuminuria (a marker for both type 1 and type 2 diabetes) develop diabetic nephropathy.

Diabetes: Retinol Complications

Diabetic retinopathy is a vascular complication of diabetes. It is the most common cause of new cases of blindness in adults ages 20 to 74. Initially, the condition causes few symptoms. However, as diabetic neuropathy progresses, patients may begin to experience blurred vision, floaters, and decreased night vision. The condition affects both eyes and can progress to blindness if not treated. Other eye disorders, such as cataracts, are also more common in those with diabetes.

Screening:
Individuals with type 1 diabetics should be screened for diabetic retinopathy within five years of diagnosis. Individuals with type 2 diabetes should be screened for diabetic neuropathy after initial diagnosis. Subsequent

to initial screening, individuals with both types of diabetes should have yearly exams or exams every two to three years if one or more yearly exam was normal.

Treatment:
Individuals with diabetic retinopathy should receive prompt referral to an ophthalmologist for laser photocoagulation therapy to prevent vision loss.

Diabetes: Neuropathic Complications

Screening:
Individuals with type 1 and type 2 diabetes should be screened for distal symmetric polyneuropathy at initial diagnosis and every year with pinprick, vibration sensation, and 10-g mono-filament testing. Individuals who have had type 1 diabetes for more than five years and individuals newly diagnosed with type 2 diabetes should be screened for autonomic neuropathy. Cardiovascular autonomic neuropathy is characterized by tachycardia (>100 beats per minute at rest) and orthostatic hypotension. Gastrointestinal neuropathies (such as gastroparesis and esophageal enteropathy) may present as constipation alternating with diarrhea. Genitourinary neuropathy may cause erectile dysfunction. A comprehensive foot examination should be performed, including screening for peripheral arterial disease with ankle-brachial index.

Education:
All patients must be taught about foot care and to examine their feet. The importance of wearing protective shoes should be stressed.

Treatment:
It is essential that the patient maintain stable glucose levels and stop smoking. Drug treatments include tricyclic antidepressants (amitriptyline, nortriptyline, and imipramine); anticonvulsants (gabapentin, carbamazepine, and pregabalin); 5-hydroxytryptamine and norepinephrine uptake inhibitors (duloxetine); and substance P inhibitor (capsaicin cream). Other treatments specific to the neuropathy (such as penile implants) are administered.

Diabetes: Cardiovascular Complications

Control of hypertension:
Patients should be screened for hypertension. If the patient is hypertensive, treatment is necessary to lower blood pressure to less than 140/80 (preferably less than 130/80).

Lipid management:
Lifestyle modifications include diet changes and increased exercise. Statin therapy is indicated for individuals with overt cardiovascular disease (CVD) and for individuals older than age 40 without CVD but with other risk factors. Lower-risk patients should have statin therapy if low-density lipoprotein (LDL) cholesterol is greater than 100 mg/dL or if multiple risk factors are present. Statin is optional with CVD if LDL is less than 70 mg/dL.

Antiplatelet agents:
Acetylsalicylic acid (ASA) at a dosage of 75 to 162 mg daily is recommended. However, the treatment is not recommended for those younger than 30 years of age. Combination therapy with clopidogrel is recommended if CVD is severe.

Smoking cessation:
No patient should smoke. Counseling and intervention should be provided.

Coronary heart disease screening:
A combination of ASA, statin, and an angiotensin-converting enzyme (ACE) inhibitor may be used to reduce the risk of acute cardiovascular events. Metformin and thiazolidinedione should not be used by those treated for congestive heart failure.

Environmental Allergens

<u>Eliminating, or at least reducing, exposure to allergens is necessary for the control of asthma.</u>
Eliminating or reducing exposure to environmental allergens can dramatically decrease symptoms' severity. Decreasing the severity of symptoms can improve the patient's quality of life. Some patients react to animal dander. To control animal dander, it may be necessary to remove the pet from the home or at least from the patient's bedroom. Air filters placed over bedroom vents can help control air circulation. Dust mites can be controlled by encasing mattresses and pillowcases in allergen-proof covers. The number of dust mites can be decreased by removing carpeting. Humidity in the home should be less than 50 percent. Insects, mold, and fungi should be controlled. In extreme cases, a person with asthma should limit his or her exposure to the outside environment, especially during times of high pollen count or increased smog.

Nonviolent Psychological Crisis

Older adults, especially those in nursing homes, must deal with many stressful situations. Older adults are just as likely to suffer from psychiatric and psychological problems as younger adults. However, older adults (especially those older than 70) are much less likely to seek the help that might prevent a psychological crisis. It is the subjective response to stress that precipitates a crisis, not the stressful event itself. Many older adults cope well with changes in their lives, but change places some older adults at increased risk for psychological crisis. People with depression, chronic illness, impaired cognition, extended bereavement, and substance abuse are at highest risk. A major life change also places individuals at increased risk for nonviolent psychological crisis.

The four categories of factors that contribute to <u>crisis</u> include
- <u>Biological</u> (illness, sensory deficits, and impaired mobility);
- <u>Environmental</u> (decreased income, retirement, and change in residence);
- <u>Psychological</u> (bereavement and cognitive impairment); and
- <u>Sociocultural</u> (role change).

<u>Managing Nonviolent Psychological Crisis</u>
Psychological crisis can be difficult to diagnose. Older adults often seek help for nonspecific physical ailments (such as headache or upset stomach) rather than specifically for anxiety or depression. When assessing an older adult, a history should always be taken. Taking a history of the complaint can bring out information that may indicate stress. The assessment should also include screening for depression because depression is highly correlated with crisis. The Geriatric Depression Scale (GDS) is used to screen for depression in older adults. Bereavement and substance abuse may also precipitate a crisis. Older adults faced with loss of memory often become very frightened and anxious. Older adults faced with changes in role experience stress. Intervention aims at reducing or eliminating stressors when possible. Older adults may benefit from cognitive-behavioral psychotherapy that teaches coping skills. Engagement in social or recreational activities may alleviate stress. In some cases, antidepressant drugs may be indicated. During treatment, the patient should be assisted to develop both short-term goals (take a one-hour nap in the afternoon, for example) and long-term goals (such as to learn relaxation techniques) to reduce stress.

Patient Death

Kübler-Ross: Model of Grieving

Elisabeth Kübler-Ross developed a model of grieving. Her model is commonly referred to as The Five Stages of Grief. She describes five distinct stages in the grieving process. Kübler-Ross postulated that people go through these stages in dealing with a tragedy, such as a terminal illness or death of a loved one. Kübler-Ross raised awareness of the need to treat individuals dealing with a terminal illness with compassion. The five stages of grief outlined by Kübler-Ross are denial, anger, bargaining, depression, and acceptance. A person may not go through every stage. The model has been criticized as having several flaws. There is little empirical research to support it. In addition, the model does not take into account how the patient's situation can affect the stages.

Five Stages of Grief
- Denial: Denial is a defense. Patients and their families may be resistive to information and unable to accept the fact of dying or impairment. They may be stunned, immobile, or detached. Patients may be unable to respond appropriately. They may not remember what is said to them and repeatedly ask the same questions.
- Anger: As reality becomes clear, patient and their families may react with pronounced anger directed inward or outward. Patients, especially women, may blame themselves, and self-anger may lead to severe depression and guilt. They may assume that they are to blame because of some personal action. Outward anger, more common in men, may be expressed as overt hostility.
- Bargaining: Bargaining involves if-then thinking (often directed at a deity). For example, a patient may think "If I go to church every day, then God will prevent this." The patient or family may change doctors, trying to change the outcome.
- Depression: As the patient and family begin to accept the loss, they may become depressed and overwhelmed with sadness. They may feel that no

one understands. They may be tearful or cry and may withdraw or ask to be left alone.
- Acceptance: This final stage represents a form of resolution and often occurs outside of the medical environment months after the diagnosis. Patients are able to accept death, dying, or incapacity. Families are able to resume their normal activities and lose the constant preoccupation with their loved one. They are able to think of the person without severe pain.

Dying Patient: Family Support

Families of dying patients often do not receive adequate support from nursing staff members, who feel unprepared for dealing with their grief and unsure of how to provide comfort. However, families may be in desperate need of this support. Before death the nurse should stay with the family and sit quietly, allowing them to talk, cry, or interact if they desire. The nurse should avoid platitudes such as "His suffering will be over soon."

The nurse should avoid judgmental reactions to what family members say or do and realize that anger, fear, guilt, and irrational behavior are normal responses to acute grief and stress. The nurse should display a caring attitude by touching the patient and encouraging family members to do the same. Touching the hands, arms, or shoulders of family members can provide comfort, but follow the cues of the family. Finally, the nurse should provide referrals to support groups if needed.

Patient Death: Family Support

At the time of death, the nurse should reassure the family that all measures have been taken to ensure the patient's comfort. The nurse should express personal feeling of loss. The nurse should provide information about what is happening during the dying process, explaining death rales and Cheyne-Stokes respirations, for example. The family members should be alerted to the patient's imminent death if they are not present. The family should be assisted in contacting clergy or spiritual advisors. The nurse should respect the feelings and needs of the spouse, children, and other family. After death, the nurse should encourage family members to stay with the patient as long as they wish to say goodbye. The nurse should assist the family to make arrangements, such as contacting the funeral home. If an autopsy is required, the nurse should discuss it with the family and explain when it will take place. If the patient's organs are being donated, the nurse should assist the family to make arrangements. The family members should be encouraged to grieve and express emotions.

End of Life: Physical Changes

There are a number of physical changes associated with the end of life. These changes are sensory, circulatory, respiratory, muscular, urinary, and integumentary.

- Sensory: Patients have reduced sensation of touch and pain, blurring of vision, and loss of blink reflex. Hearing is usually the last of the senses to fail, so the patient should be communicated with in a way he or she will understand during the dying process.
- Circulatory: Tachycardia is followed by bradycardia and weakening of the pulse with irregular rhythm. Blood pressure decreases.
- Respiratory: Tachypnea progresses to Cheyne-Stokes respirations. The patient is unable to cough or clear secretions, so rattling may be heard. Breathing becomes increasingly irregular with terminal gasping.
- Muscular: The patient loses the ability to move, talk, and swallow. The gag reflex is lost. The jaw begins to sag,

and occasional jerking may be seen if the patient is receiving narcotics.
- Urinary: Urinary output decreases. The patient is incontinent and then unable to urinate.
- Integumentary: The skin becomes cold and clammy. Mottling and cyanosis may appear. The skin takes on a waxy appearance.

Regard Individual Beliefs and Traditions

Individual beliefs and traditions regarding death vary widely, and these affect how the patient and his or her family deal with the end of life. The nurse should discuss these issues with the patient and/or family members in order to ensure that their needs are met. Those with strong spiritual beliefs may want spiritual advisors (such as priests, shamans, ministers, or monks) present to provide support or perform rituals. People who have no belief in an afterlife may face death with resolution or may be frightened at the thought of the total end of their existence. Individuals who believe in reincarnation may find comfort in the thought of their rebirth but may also fear karma for the mistakes they made in this life. Some people believe in a loving God, while others believe in a vengeful God. Some individuals may feel that they will be in a loving place after death, while others fear they will suffer torment for their sins. The nurse should remain supportive and allow patients and families to express their feelings, fears, and concerns.

Grief and Loss

Older adults must cope with almost continuous grief and loss, including primary losses (spouse, friends, and family) and secondary losses (such as companionship and assistance). As losses accumulate, the older adult may become overwhelmed with grief and unable to cope. Patients may grieve the following losses: body image (physical and psychological as physical condition deteriorates), spouse/partner/friends (through death or distance), self-identity and self-esteem (as roles change), possessions (if people move from a home to an assisted living or other long-term care facility), financial stability (as income decreases and expenses increase), dignity (as others care for the person), independence (as the person is forced to rely on others for assistance), mental acuity, and life itself (including that of significant others). The older adult's ability to cope with grief and loss and find hope depends upon his or her support system, health status, mental status, and belief system.

Depression and Anger

Older adults may exhibit a number of different psychological responses to loss. These responses may interfere with their ability to function and can interfere with medical care. Depression is the most common response of older adults to loss. Patients may become increasingly withdrawn and sad. This response puts them at risk for suicide. They may feel that life is futile and refuse medical care.

Anger is also a response to loss. Some older adults focus on the unfairness of their situation and become mired in anger, often antagonizing friends and family and behaving belligerently. They may refuse to cooperate or actively resist care. These individuals may blame the doctors, nurses, and family for their circumstances and find fault with almost everything and everyone. Their relationships often suffer as a result of this behavior.

Confusion, Dependence and Passivity

Older adults coping with loss may exhibit confusion, dependence, and passivity. The frequency and speed of changes and loss may overwhelm the older adult, resulting in increasing confusion. This is especially true if the person has even a mild degree of cognitive impairment. However, even those without dementia may exhibit the same symptoms, such as forgetting to take medications, missing appointments, and confusing directions. The person may appear disoriented. In response to stress, some older adults become very dependent on others often to the point of being clingy and demanding of attention. They may call family members constantly or demand attention to receive reassurance. They may become very distressed if asked to make independent decisions. Some older adults begin to believe that they have no control and become very passive, allowing others to make decisions in matters concerning them. These patients are not engaged in their life or health concerns, deferring to doctors, nurses, and family members.

Change of Residence

Change of residence for an older adult may involve a move to an apartment, assisted living facility, or nursing home. These changes can be very disorienting for the older adult who must cope with a new environment and new people. The older adult must also cope with the grief of losing former associations and personal belongings. If at all possible, the older adult should be included in plans prior to a move. The move is made easier if the older adult is taken to visit the facility and allowed to meet some of the staff or people there. Even in very restricted environments, such as nursing homes, patients are usually allowed a few personal belongings, such as family pictures and a few items of clothing. Personal items can provide some comfort to older adults in new surroundings. Patients whose family and friends visit may cope better than those with no support system.

Loss of a Spouse

The loss of a spouse can be devastating to the survivor, who often responds with severe depression and sometimes becomes suicidal. The response may depend on the quality of the relationship. If the partners had a poor or abusive relationship, the surviving spouse may feel some relief but also anger and guilt and may have difficulty assuming more independence. Because women tend to live longer than men, there are more widows than widowers. As some retirement benefits decrease when a spouse dies, women often lose a significant amount of their income when the spouse dies. Women often grieve more openly than men because men feel constrained by societal expectations. However, men may feel great loss. Men are often better able to afford to pay for assistance with chores previously done by a spouse, such as cooking and cleaning. Divorce, which is becoming more common with older adults, can result in similar effects.

Loss of Independence and Autonomy

The loss of independence and autonomy associated with aging is profoundly disturbing to many older adults. Losing the ability to live independently increases overall dependency on others, especially if older adults must live with family members or in a long-term care facility. Losing the ability to drive can prevent older adults from shopping and engaging in social activities. This loss may be devastating to some individuals and may increase symptoms of depression. Many people, especially males, do not willingly give up driving and are forced to do so because of safety concerns by family or physicians. These individuals may become very angry and resentful. Role reversal may occur as older adults' children become their care providers and increasingly make decisions for them. This may cause conflicts that are draining to both parties, and some older adults become increasingly dependent and demanding. Assistance with instrumental activities of daily living (IADLs) and activities of daily living (ADLs) is often necessary, but older adults who want to remain autonomous may resist the help.

Sexuality

Human sexuality is important to adults of all ages. Older adults need and often crave intimacy with others, including sexual intimacy. Health-care providers should address this issue directly with their older patients as patients may be embarrassed or reluctant to ask questions. Although the issue of sexual intimacy in older adults may be uncomfortable, nurses should not avoid the topic because of personal anxiety. Further, the nurse should respect different attitudes and behavior. Assessment should be done in private, ensuring confidentiality. Questioning should progress from general topics ("Do you have a good relationship with your partner?") to more specific questions related to sexual issues ("Is intercourse uncomfortable for you?"). Older adults may need to know how to deal with physical or environmental limitations. Some older adults engage in sexual behavior that puts them at increased risk of human immunodeficiency virus (HIV) or sexually transmitted diseases (STDs). Discussing sexual issues provides an opportunity for education and counseling.

Sexuality and Cardiovascular Considerations

Older adults with cardiovascular disease (such as myocardial infarction and angina) may be very anxious and fearful about sexual activity, but the risks associated with sexual activity are very low, and most heart recovery programs encourage exercise. There are a number of things to keep in mind. The participants should be well rested, so morning or after a nap may be the best time for sexual activity. The participants should wait one to three hours after eating before engaging in sexual activity. The couple should use whatever position is comfortable for them. If pressure on the chest is an issue, the couple may feel less anxious in side-lying positions. The couple should engage in foreplay so that the heart rate increases and strengthens in preparation for sexual intercourse. If one of the participants is taking nitroglycerin for angina, he or she should take the medication prior to sexual activity to prevent angina.

Sexuality and Chronic Health Problems

Chronic health problems that affect stamina and mobility may pose challenges for older adults engaging in sexual activity. There are several actions that can make things easier. The participant with the health problem should be well rested and engage in sexual activities at the time of day when he or she has the most energy. This is usually in the morning. A person with chronic pain should engage in sexual activity when pain medication is at peak effectiveness. It should be noted that orgasm releases endorphins that may relieve pain for hours after sexual activity. Taking a warm bath prior to sexual activity may relax the muscles and relieve stiffness. It may take some experimentation for the couple to find a position that is comfortable for both. Males with Foley catheters can fold the catheter up against the shaft of the penis and apply a condom to secure it. Females with Foley catheters can position the catheter upward and away from the vagina. The couple may engage in manual and/or oral stimulation.

Sexuality among Homosexuals

The gay rights movement began in 1969. Therefore, many older adults came to maturity at a time when prejudice and discrimination against gays and lesbians was overt, tolerated, and sometimes legislated. Because of this, many older adults are not open about their sexuality and may be reluctant to discuss their concerns. The nurse can open the lines of communication by asking patients directly if they have sex with the same gender while showing respect for the individual. Since marriage between gays and lesbians is legal in only a few states, their partners usually lack the legal status conferred on spouses. Nurses and other

health-care providers should respect the bond between two people even if it is not a traditional relationship. Nurses should encourage expressions of intimacy between the partners. Most gay and lesbian organizations are geared toward younger members, so there is a dearth of social services aimed at the older population.

Intimacy in Nursing Homes

The need for intimacy doesn't end when older adults enter nursing homes, but there can be many obstacles to the expression of intimacy in nursing homes. The patient may have serious health problems that limit physical intimacy. Many rooms house two patients, and lack of privacy is an issue. Most facilities have only single beds available for patients. Even if the patient is in a private room, staff members are in and out of rooms frequently, interfering with privacy. Nurses and other staff may have stereotypical negative attitudes toward older adults and sexuality. Every effort should be made to overcome obstacles and allow partners/spouses private time with patients. Even if sexual intercourse is not possible, the partners can hold and caress each other and express their caring. Curtains can be drawn to provide privacy or a notice can be placed on the door ("Family time").

Pets

Many older adults, especially those who are essentially homebound, consider pets to be members of the family. A pet may be an older adult's only companion. Dog owners tend to walk more, which improves mobility and maintains muscle strength. Pet ownership can have both physical and psychological benefits. Pet ownership has been found to lower blood pressure, increase self-esteem, and improve quality of life. Some animal rescue organizations (such as the SPCA) offer low-cost adoptions for seniors, and some food banks now offer pet food for those with pets.

Entering a pet-restricted facility can be wrenching for older adults, and some refuse medical or assistive care in order to stay with their pets. Older adults who must relinquish pets should be assisted to find suitable homes for them. Ideally, the new owner would bring the animal for visits. Increasing numbers of facilities are allowing animals to visit. Animals should be bathed within 24 hours of a visit to a nursing home or other facility. They should be leashed or caged and under the control of a handler.

Addiction

Alcohol Addiction

All patients should be assessed for alcohol addiction as part of the initial physical exam. If there are health indications (abnormal liver function tests, falls, or insomnia) or social indications (family problems, divorce, or job loss) subsequent assessments should be made. There are numerous self-assessment screening tools used to measure drinking. About 33 percent of older adult alcoholics began drinking at an older age, often in response to depression. Social drinking is common in retirement facilities. Studies indicate that there may be some health benefits to the consumption of small amounts of wine, but alcohol often interacts with drugs and this can lead to complications. Therefore, the patient should not drink until the physician has reviewed the patient's medications and determined that it is safe. If the patient has a problem with alcohol, the nurse should discuss the assessment with the patient. The patient should be informed of the health consequences of drinking. The patient should be provided with information about resources (such as Alcoholics Anonymous and alcohol rehabilitation programs).

Prescription Drug Addictions

Abuse of prescription drugs includes taking a lower dose than prescribed, taking a higher dose than prescribed, or taking the drugs erratically. Older adults are particularly vulnerable to abuse of prescription drugs because of easy access. Approximately a third of all prescriptions are written for older adults. Many older adults are isolated and have infrequent contact with health-care providers. For these reasons, symptoms of prescription drug abuse (such as confusion, falls, or lethargy) may be overlooked or attributed to health conditions, such as Alzheimer's disease. People who abuse alcohol often abuse prescription drugs as well, so assessment of alcohol abuse should also include assessment for drug abuse. Patients who abuse drugs may see a number of different physicians to obtain prescriptions. Narcotic analgesics (taken to control chronic pain) and central nervous system depressants (taken to reduce anxiety and improve sleep) are the most commonly abused prescription drugs. Patients often deny abuse of drugs even though the evidence of abuse is clear. Treatment may include behavioral therapy, medications to relieve withdrawal symptoms, and 12-step or other recovery programs.

Long-Term Substance Abuse

Many people with substance abuse (alcohol or drugs) are reluctant to disclose this information. However, there are a number of indicators suggestive of long-term substance abuse. Physical signs of long-term substance abuse include needle tracks on the arms or legs, burns on the fingers or lips, abnormally dilated or constricted pupils, watery eyes, slurred speech/slow speech, lack of coordination, gait instability, tremors, repeated sniffing, nasal irritation, persistent cough, weight loss, and dysrhythmia. Other symptoms include pallor; puffiness of the face; odor of alcohol/marijuana on the clothing or breath; labile emotions (including mood swings, agitation, and anger); inappropriate, impulsive, and/or risky behavior; difficulty concentrating/short term memory loss; disorientation/ confusion;

blackouts; insomnia or excessive sleeping; and lack of personal hygiene. An individual abusing drugs or alcohol may be unreliable and lie or miss appointments.

Tobacco Addiction

Approximately 10 percent of adults older than 65 use tobacco (primarily cigarettes). Many more are former smokers. Older adult smokers are at particular risk for smoking-related diseases because they often have smoked for more than 40 years and are usually heavy smokers. Smoking is the cause of 90 percent of chronic obstructive pulmonary disease cases. Smokers are twice as likely as nonsmokers to die from stroke or heart attack. Smoking reduces life expectancy by 13 to 15 years, so patients of any age should be advised to quit completely. Quitting smoking can prolong life and improve the quality of life. Simply reducing the amount of tobacco used has little health benefit, and use usually increases again after a time. Many long-term smokers have numerous health problems related to smoking. Smokers may be extremely resistant to quitting in spite of the health risks because of tobacco's addictive qualities. Patients who abuse other substances (alcohol or drugs) are more likely to fall asleep while smoking than patients who do not abuse other substances and are more likely to suffer burns as a consequence.

Gambling Addiction

Older adults often find it easy to gamble with the prevalence of lotteries, casinos, and Internet gambling sites. Older adults may turn to gambling as an outlet for frustration or stress and may not understand the dynamics of addiction before they have squandered their savings. Because of the difficulty older adults have in finding employment, they may not be able to replace the money that they lost, resulting in increasing poverty and stress. Older adults who get into debt through gambling may argue about the habit with family or friends.

Older adults with cognitive impairment may not completely understand the implications of losing money gambling. Gambling problems may be difficult to identify, because older adults may hide their addiction because of embarrassment. They are often reluctant to seek counseling to help them stop gambling. Signs of gambling include an increased focus on gambling to the exclusion of other activities; physical problems such as headaches, increased anxiety, depression, bowel and bladder problems, and constant tiredness; and financial concerns and lack of basic needs (such as food and clothing).

Sex Addiction

Sex addiction occurs when people become fixated on sex, arousal, and thrill seeking. The act of sex becomes more important than intimacy. This addiction often causes people to seek sexual relations with multiple partners (sometimes younger), including prostitutes. Sex addiction may also take the form of masturbation in response to Internet pornography or inappropriate behavior, such as masturbating in public or exposing oneself. Sex addiction that involves multiple partners increases the danger of both getting and spreading sexually transmitted diseases (STDs). While it does not cause sex addiction, Viagra (and other such drugs) can fuel sex addiction in males. Indications of sex addiction include increasing need for sexual stimulation; inability to control sexual urges; engaging in high-risk sexual activities (such as contact with prostitutes); utilizing sexual fantasies to cope with stress; mood swings; and neglecting social obligations, family, and friends. Most people with sex addiction are reluctant to discuss their disorder. The subject should be raised with individuals with STDs or those found engaging in inappropriate behavior. The disorder is treated with behavioral therapy.

Recreational Drug Use

Illicit recreational drug use by older adults in the United States is expected to increase 300 percent between 2001 and 2020. Currently, the incidence of recreational drug use among older adults is a relatively low 1.7 percent (up from 1 percent 10 years ago). However, this percentage is expected to increase dramatically as more long-term users from the baby boomer generation enter older age. Adding to the increase is the fact that methadone programs and better treatment for human immunodeficiency virus/acquired immune deficiency syndrome (HIV/AIDS) have prolonged the lives of illicit drug users, many of whom in the past would not have lived to an older age. The stress of dealing with aging and chronic illness causes some older adults to turn to recreational drugs to reduce stress or relieve symptoms. Marijuana, which is the most frequently abused recreational drug, is frequently taken for "health" reasons. Marijuana may impair short-term memory, executive functioning, and attention. Treatment for drug use includes behavioral therapy and 12-step programs. Programs geared toward older adults are usually more successful in treating this age group.

Domestic Violence

According to the guidelines of the Family Violence Prevention Fund, all adult patients should be assessed for *domestic violence*. Individuals of all ages and backgrounds can be victims of domestic abuse. Abuse does not stop because couples age. Females are the most frequent victims of domestic abuse. However, there are increasing reports of male victims of domestic violence, both in heterosexual and homosexual relationships. The person doing the assessment should be knowledgeable about domestic violence and be aware of risk factors and danger signs. The interview should be *conducted in private*. The nurse's office and the bathrooms and examining rooms in the facility should have information about domestic violence posted prominently. Brochures and information should be made available to each patient. Patients may present with a variety of physical complaints, such as headache, pain, palpitations, numbness, or pelvic pain. Victims of domestic violence are often depressed and may appear suicidal. They may be isolated from friends and family. Victims of domestic violence often exhibit fear of their spouse or partner and may give an explanation inconsistent with their injuries.

Injuries

There are a number of characteristic injuries that may indicate domestic violence, including ruptured eardrum; rectal/genital injury (burns, bites, or trauma); scrapes and bruises about the neck, face, head, trunk, arms; and cuts, bruises, and fractures of the face. The pattern of injuries associated with domestic violence is also often distinctive. The bathing-suit pattern involves injuries on parts of body that are usually covered with clothing as the perpetrator inflicts damage but hides evidence of abuse. Head and neck injuries (50%) are also common. Abusive injuries (rarely attributable to accidents) are common and include bites, bruises, rope and cigarette burns, and welts in the outline of weapons (belt marks). Bilateral injuries of arms/legs are often seen with domestic abuse. Defensive injuries are indicative of abuse.

Defensive injuries to the back of the body are often incurred as the victim crouches on the floor face down while being attacked. The soles of the feet may be injured from kicking at perpetrator. The ulnar aspect of hand or palm may be injured from blocking blows.

Victim Identification
- Inquiry: The patient should be asked if any physical, sexual, or psychological abuse has taken place.

- Interview: The person may be anxious or fearful. The person should be asked if he or she is afraid for his or her life.
- Question: If abuse is reported, it's critical to ask if the person is in immediate danger or if the abuser is on the premises.
- Validate: The interviewer should offer support and reassurance, telling the patient the abuse is not his or her fault.
- Give information: The interviewer should state that violence has a tendency to escalate. The interviewer should provide information about safety planning. If the patient wants to file a complaint with the police, the interviewer should provide assistance.
- Make referrals: Information about state, local, and national organizations should be provided along with telephone numbers and contact numbers for domestic violence shelters.
- Document: Legal, legible, and lengthy records should be kept with a complete description of any traumatic injuries. A body map may be used to indicate sites of injury.

Elder Abuse

Elder abuse may be difficult to diagnose, especially if the person is cognitively impaired. Active abuse is intentional (such as hitting) while passive abuse occurs without intention. Signs and symptoms of elder abuse can include fearfulness, disparities between patient and caregiver reports of injuries, evidence of old or repeated injuries, poor hygiene, poor dental care, bed sores, and malnutrition. Furthermore, the caregiver may be unduly concerned with costs and may appear unsupportive. The caregiver may be reluctant to allow the patient to communicate privately with the nurse. Diagnosis includes a careful history and physical exam, including direct questioning of the patient about abuse.

Treatment includes attending to the patient's injuries and physical needs. Referral should be made to adult protective services as indicated. Reporting laws regarding elder abuse vary somewhat from one state to another, but all states have laws regarding elder abuse, and most states require mandatory reporting to adult protective services by health-care workers.

Risk of Elder Abuse

Age and disability increase the risks of elder abuse. People older than age 80 are more than twice as likely to suffer abuse as younger adults. Abuse takes place in both the home and in institutions. At home, older adults with dementia are often abused by family members. Caregivers often lose patience and become frustrated, especially if the patient's behavior is belligerent, combative, or disruptive. Five to fourteen percent of those with dementia are victims of elder abuse. One to three percent of individuals in the general population are victims of elder abuse. Elder abuse of individuals with dementia can be very difficult to diagnose, as the patient is usually unable to report the abuse. In fact, even older adults who are not cognitively impaired may be afraid to report abuse because they depend on their abuser to care for them. Older adults who are dependent on caregivers for assistance with activities of daily living (ADLs) are particularly at risk for abuse and neglect. Abusers often suffer from depression and/or substance abuse and may be financially dependent on the victim.

Physical And Psychological Abuse

There are a number of different types of elder abuse. Physical abuse is an active form of abuse (a type of domestic violence). It is almost always associated with psychological abuse. Older adults may suffer various types of assaults, including slapping, punching, kicking, hair pulling, and shoving. The physical abuse of an older adult is often committed by a family member (often an adult child) or other caregiver. Caregivers may make frequent threats to hit the older adult if he or she doesn't cooperate with the caregiver's plan. The caregiver may brandish a weapon. In addition, the caretaker may tell the person to commit suicide. Ongoing intimidation may make cause terror and anxiety. Sometimes, caregivers threaten to injure pets or family members, increasing the patient's fear. Patients may be forcibly confined, forced into seclusion, and/or force-fed to the point that they choke on food. Physical symptoms are consistent with domestic abuse. Psychological symptoms include anxiety, paranoia, insomnia, low self-esteem, avoidance of eye contact, and nervousness in the presence of the caregiver, who is often reluctant to leave the patient alone.

Financial Abuse

As older adults become unable to manage their own financial affairs, they become increasingly vulnerable to financial abuse. This is especially true if the adult has cognitive impairment or physical impairments that impair mobility. Financial abuse includes outright stealing of property or persuading the patient to give away possessions, forcing the individual to sign away property, emptying the individual's bank and savings accounts, stealing the individual's credit cards, convincing the individual to invest money in fraudulent schemes, and taking money from the individual for home renovations that are not done. Indications of financial abuse may be unpaid bills, unusual activity at ATMs, unusual credit activity, inadequate funds to meet needs, disappearance of items from the home, change in the provision of a will, and deferring to caregivers regarding financial affairs. Family members or caregivers may move permanently into the patient's home and take over without sharing costs.

Abuse and Neglect of Basic Needs

Neglect of basic needs is a common problem of older adults who live alone or with reluctant or incapable caregivers. In some cases, passive neglect may occur because an elderly spouse is trying to take care of a patient and is unable to provide the care needed. Active neglect is intentional and reflects a lack of caring. Active neglect may border on negligence and abuse. Indications of neglect include lack of assistive devices needed for mobility (such as cane or walker); lack of needed glasses or hearing aids; poor dental hygiene and dental care and/or missing dentures; inadequate food/fluid/nutrition, resulting in weight loss; inappropriate and unkempt clothing (for example, the lack of a sweater or coat during the winter and dirty or torn clothing); and a dirty, messy environment. In addition, the patient may be left unattended for prolonged periods of time (sometimes confined to a bed or chair) or left in soiled or urine-/feces-stained clothing.

Sexual Abuse

Sexual abuse of older adults occurs when the person receiving sexual attention is forced to participate or unable to consent to sexual intimacy. Patients may be unable to consent to sexual activity due to cognitive impairment or other illness. Types of sexual abuse include physical (fondling, kissing, and rape); emotional (exhibitionism); and verbal (sexual harassment, using obscene language, and threatening). Women in their seventies or eighties who are confined to nursing homes are the most frequent targets of sexual abuse. Sexual abuse may also occur in home environments, but it is harder to detect. Most abusers of women in nursing homes are males older than age 80 who reside in the same nursing home. The most common form of abuse is sexualized kissing and fondling of the genitals. Older adults do behave sexually and in some cases what appears to be abuse between residents is, in fact, consensual sexual activity. Caregivers have raped or otherwise sexually abused patients, and this exercise of power over another person is always illegal abuse.

Exercise

General Guidelines

Exercises should be tailored for the individual older adult. Warm-up exercises should be part of any exercise program and should be performed before participation in sports activities. Warm-up exercises increase circulation and muscle elasticity and prevent injury. Warm-up exercises should begin slowly and systematically involve all parts of the body. There are three types of warm-up: passive, general bodywide, and specific stretching motions. Passive warm-up may include a massage or a warm shower. General bodywide warm-ups may include brisk walking. Specific stretching motions should be bilateral and static. It's important to stretch and warm up all muscles, but special attention should be paid to the muscles most used in the activity. Exercise should be low to moderate in intensity to prevent injury. The duration of exercise should be increased gradually to 30 or more minutes daily (or three 10-minute periods) with a goal of daily exercise.

Strengthening Exercises

Older adults may benefit from strengthening exercises to improve both strength and mobility. Many facilities offer special exercise programs for older adults. The exercises follow a progression:

Isometric exercises are done with the muscle and limb in static position with no movement of the joint or lengthening of the muscle. The muscle is contracted against resistance. Isotonic exercises include movement of the joint during exercise (such as walking and weight lifting) and both shortening and lengthening of the muscles through eccentric or concentric contractions. Isotonic refers to tension, so the tension is constant during shortening and lengthening of the muscle. Isokinetic exercises make use of machines (such as stationary bicycles) to control the rate and extent of contraction as well as the range of motion. Both speed and resistance can be set, so the patient is limited by the settings of the machine.

Cardiovascular Conditioning and Endurance Training

Because cardiovascular and respiratory fitness can decrease rapidly with inactivity, it is important to engage in cardiovascular conditioning and endurance training after injury or illness. The type of cardiovascular exercises recommended will depend upon the site of injury and the phase of healing. If there is an injury of a lower extremity, then non–weight-bearing exercises (for example, swimming, weight lifting, or upper-body cycling) may be indicated. If there is an injury to an upper extremity, then weight-bearing exercises (such as climbing stairs, running, aerobics, or use of elliptical machines) are more appropriate. Cardiac rehabilitation focuses on the whole body. In all cases, the type of cardiovascular conditioning should be tailored to the individual.

Aquatic Exercise

Aquatic exercise can be very beneficial to older adults. Aquatic exercise can effectively increase range of motion of the arms and legs and improve balance by strengthening the trunk and abdomen. Immersion in water causes a number of physiological effects unrelated to the exercises. Physiological changes include increased cardiac and intrapulmonary blood volume with increases in pressure in the right atrium and increased volume at left ventricular diastole. In addition, there is increased stroke volume and overall cardiac output. Concurrently, there is a reduction in peripheral circulation and lung expansion, decreasing vital capacity. Heart rate often remains unchanged or remains significantly lower than when doing similar exercises outside of the water. This effect depends on the depth of the water and speed of exercise. Resistance in water increases with depth of immersion up to about the middle of the body. After this point, buoyancy counterbalances resistance. Exercising in water at waist level results in a similar heart rate and consumption of oxygen as exercising out of the water.

Kegel Exercises

Kegel exercises work the pelvic floor muscles. These exercises are used to strengthen the periurethral and pelvic muscles in order to increase control of urination and defecation. These exercises can be used to improve urinary and fecal incontinence. The basic exercises involve tightening the muscles three to four times daily for about three seconds and then relaxing for the same period. The exercises should be repeated about 10 times, gradually increasing the time tightening the muscles to 5 to 10 seconds. Isolating the right muscles to tighten is important. Tightening the stomach, leg, or other muscles will not work the pelvic floor muscles. People should not hold their breath during the exercises because this may tighten other muscles. There are three methods to check that the pelvic floor muscles are flexing:

- Stop the flow of urine in the middle of urination.
- Pull in the anus as though trying to stop from passing flatus.
- In the supine position, place a finger inside the vagina and squeeze as if trying to stop the flow of urine. Tightness should be felt.

How to Perform Kegel Exercises
Kegel exercises strengthen the muscles of the pelvic floor. The urethra, rectum, and vagina all open through the pelvic-floor muscles, which support the pelvic organs. Holding the

breath or tightening the abdominal muscles or buttock muscles should be avoided during pelvic-floor exercises.

- Procedure: Tighten and squeeze the muscles around the rectum, vagina, and urethra and try to lift them inside as though trying to stop from passing gas and urine. Hold the tension for the prescribed period of time and relax. Rest a few seconds and repeat the exercise.
- Schedule: Exercises should be done at least three times each day. They may be done while lying down or sitting.
- 1–2 weeks: Tighten the muscles for 1 second and relax for 5. Repeat the procedure 10 times. Then, tighten 5 seconds and relax 10. Repeat the procedure 10 times.
- 3–4 weeks: Tighten the muscles for 5 to10 seconds and relax for 10. Repeat the procedure 20 times.
- 5–6 weeks: Tighten the muscles for 8–10 seconds and relax for 10. Repeat the procedure 20 times.

Urinary Incontinence and Bowel Issues

The Knack: Control Urinary Incontinence

The Knack is the use of precisely timed muscle contractions to prevent urination due to stress incontinence. It is "the knack" of squeezing up before bearing down. The knack is a preventive use of Kegel exercises. The procedure involves contracting the pelvic floor muscles immediately before and during events that usually cause stress incontinence. For example, if a woman feels that she is going to cough or sneeze, she immediately contracts the pelvic floor muscles and holds the tension until the stress event is over. This contraction provides additional support for the proximal urethra and reduces the amount of displacement that usually occurs with compromised muscle support. This technique is particularly useful if used before and during stress events, such as coughing, sneezing, lifting, standing, swinging a golf club, or laughing. Women who are taught this technique for mild to moderate urinary incontinence and use it consistently are able to decrease incontinence by 73 to 98 percent.

Nocturia

Nocturia is a condition in which an individual wakes up one or more times during the night with the need to urinate. Some authorities believe that one event per night is within normal limits. Some people have to urinate five or six times each night. In about 70 percent of cases, nocturia is related to overproduction of urine at night. Nocturia is one of the most common causes of sleep deprivation. Approximately two-thirds of those older than age 50 have nocturia. Studies have shown that nocturia involving urination more than two times each night is strongly linked to depression. The goal of treatment is to reduce urination during the night. Treatment involves medication and/or fluid management. The primary treatment for nocturia is the medication desmopressin (Stimate). This drug acts as an antidiuretic hormone that reduces volume of urine by increasing concentration. This medication allows for about five hours of undisturbed sleep. It increases the first period of sleep by about two hours. Fluid management by reducing fluids in the evening can help some people.

Overactive Bladder

Overactive bladder is a condition involving urgency, frequency, and nocturia but not incontinence. The urge to urinate may be as frequent as every 20 to 30 minutes in extreme cases. If nocturia is present, people may become sleep deprived. If overactive bladder includes incontinence, it is known as urge incontinence. The treatments are similar for overactive bladder and urge incontinence. Treatment includes drug therapy, specific exercises, behavioral modification, fluid management, and dietary changes.

Anticholinergics (antimuscarinics) such as Detrol and Ditropan relax the bladder muscle and relieve symptoms. Pelvic-floor muscle exercises include Kegel exercises and vaginal weight training as well as biofeedback or pelvic-floor electrical stimulation conducted in conjunction with the Kegel exercise program. Behavioral modification involves bladder training, including scheduled voiding with increasing time between urinations, and strategies to delay urination. Prompted urination may be needed for some people, especially those with dementia. Fluid management involves decreasing fluids in the evening while still maintaining adequate fluid intake. Reducing caffeine and other ingested bladder irritants may reduce contractions.

Bladder Retraining

Bladder retraining teaches people to control the urge to urinate. It usually takes about three months to strengthen a bladder muscle weakened from frequent urination. Frequent urination may cause a decreased urinary capacity. A short urination interval is gradually lengthened to every two to four hours during the daytime. The urge to void is resisted for increasingly longer periods of time. To start, the person keeps a bladder (or urination) diary for a week to establish a baseline frequency. An individual program is established with scheduled voiding times and goals. For example, if a person is urinating every hour, the goal might be every 80 minutes with increased output. When the urination goal is met consistently, a new goal is established. The progress is charted in the urination diary. The person is taught techniques to stop urination. For example, the person is instructed to sit on a hard seat or on a tightly rolled towel to put pressure on pelvic floor muscles and squeeze the pelvic floor muscles five times while breathing deeply and counting backwards from 50.

Bowel Retraining

Bowel retraining is a program that helps people to establish control over their bowel movements. This training involves strategies to develop a routine schedule for defecation. The individual keeps a bowel diary for a week to establish a baseline. Diet and fluid intake are modified to assure normal stool consistency. Fiber and fluid intake may be increased. The individual is instructed to eat meals at scheduled times and avoid foods that increase bowel dysfunction. A schedule for defecation is established, preferably at the same time each day and about 20 to 30 minutes after a meal. Eating stimulates the gastrocolic reflex that propels fecal material through the colon. The individual is taught Kegel exercises to strengthen muscles. A stimulus is used to promote defecation. Enemas, suppositories, or laxatives may be used to stimulate defecation in the beginning, but the goal is to decrease the use of these products. Digital stimulation or hot drinks may be used. The person keeps a record of stool consistency and evacuation.

Strategies to Prevent Constipation and Fecal Impaction

There are a number of management strategies to prevent constipation and fecal impaction. These include adding fiber to the diet in the form of bran, fresh/dried fruits, and whole grains to 20 to 35 grams per day; increasing fluids to 64 ounces each day; and exercising every day. If the individual is capable of walking, this form of exercise should be included in the regimen. Certain medications can cause constipation. If this is the case, these medications can be changed. The use of stool softeners (Colace) or bulk formers (Metamucil) may decrease fluid absorption and move stool through the colon more quickly. Overuse of laxatives can cause constipation. Careful monitoring of diet, fluids, and medical treatment, especially for irritable bowel syndrome, can aid in the management of bowel movements. Delayed toileting should be avoided. A bowel-training regimen should be followed to promote evacuation at the same time each day.

Special Issues

High Blood Pressure: Diet and Exercise

The Seventh Report of the Joint National Committee on Prevention, Detection, Evaluation, and Treatment of High Blood Pressure has recommended a number of lifestyle changes to reduce weight:

Decrease sedentary behaviors:
Long periods spent watching television, searching the Internet, playing video games, and instant messaging should be avoided. A time limit should be established to encourage physical activity.

Increase exercise and physical activity:
Everyone should engage in at least 30 minutes of exercise daily (a minimum 150 minutes/week) if possible. Walking, biking, aerobic dancing, weight lifting, tennis, and exercise and dance classes are beneficial. Group activities, such as hiking, can encourage participation.

Modify diet:
Food portions, dietary fat, and simple carbohydrates should be reduced. Snacking between meals should be avoided or healthy snacks (such as celery sticks) substituted.

Mental Aerobics

Mental aerobics are exercises that help maintain cognitive ability and memory skills. Individuals who remain active mentally have a lower incidence of Alzheimer's disease. Mental exercise may slow the progression of dementia and prompt neurogenesis (development of new neurons). Exercises should focus on right-brain, left-brain, and whole-brain stimulation. Older adults should start with simple exercises and then progress to more difficult ones. Many different types of activities can be classified as mental aerobics. The goal of these activities is to exert mental effort to "exercise" the brain. Many types of mental activity stimulate the brain including taking classes and learning new information, reading books that contain new material, solving puzzles (crossword, jigsaw, Sudoku, scrambled words, symbol sequence, and mazes); using the nondominant hand to eat, draw, comb hair, brush teeth, or write; using mnemonic devices to help facilitate short- and long-term memory; and studying a new language.

Poor Hygiene

Poor hygiene in older adults increases the risk of disease and infection. Poor hygiene is often attributable to physical impairment (such as poor vision or decreased mobility), depression, or cognitive impairment (Alzheimer's disease or substance abuse). Many older adults may require assistance with hygiene. Older adults don't need daily baths, but they should bathe two to three times weekly. Grab bars, shower or tub seats, tub mats, handheld showers, and proper heating (to avoid chilling the patient) can facilitate more frequent bathing. The use of mild soap and bath oil may help prevent drying of the skin. Individuals with dementia are often fearful of tubs and showers and may find a sponge bath or Comfort Bath with premoistened, warmed towelettes preferable. Clothing that is easy to manipulate (such as pull-on pants) and clothes with Velcro closures may make it easier for older adults to change clothes and encourage bathing. Thick-handled toothbrushes or electric toothbrushes may facilitate mouth care.

Sun Exposure

For many years, older adults were advised to protect their skin from all sun exposure in order to prevent skin damage that could lead to skin cancer. However, this behavior in conjunction with a decrease in milk drinking has resulted in an increased incidence of vitamin D deficiency in all ages. This is fueling a debate between physicians who believe that some sun exposure is warranted and others who insist that all exposure is harmful. Recent guidelines suggest that approximately 20 minutes of sun exposure daily with the arms exposed (avoiding direct sun from 10 AM to 2 PM) is a safe level of exposure and will prevent vitamin D deficiency. Sunburns should be avoided. Dark-skinned patients may tolerate more time in the sun without burning. For longer periods of time, sunscreen should be applied to all exposed areas of skin. Individuals who are fair and prone to burning must be especially careful. Skin cancers, including squamous cell carcinoma, basal cell carcinoma, and malignant melanoma, are on the rise in older adults.

International Patient Safety Goals

Gerontological nurses may work in institutions accredited by the Joint Commission, but even those in other types of practices can use the International Patient Safety Goals as a patient-care strategy that includes adhering to goals, educating support staff, and monitoring for compliance. Nurses should adhere to the following strategies: identify patients correctly (use two identifiers for medicines, blood, or blood products); read the checklist before beginning surgery (ensure correct patient, procedure, and body part); improve effective communication (establish a procedure for taking orders and reports and read back verbal/telephone orders); remove concentrated electrolytes from patient care units, especially potassium; read the surgical checklist (ensure the proper documentation is present and the necessary equipment is in working order); mark surgical site (mark the surgical site with clear identifiable markings); comply with hand-washing standards (use Centers for Disease Control guidelines for hand washing); and assess the risk of falls (eliminate fall risks).

Assistive Devices

There are many different assistive devices available for use by older adults. These include basic items (dentures, Velcro openings, elastic shoestrings, and grab bars); tools (reaching devices and special cookware, dishes, and silverware); and large pieces of equipment (oxygen tanks, wheelchairs, walkers, and commodes). Maintaining assistive devices can be difficult for older adults. The first step is to assist the person to make a comprehensive list of devices he or she uses and then prepare a checklist indicating what needs to be done for maintenance. This process also helps the nurse to evaluate the need for assistive devices. Different types of devices require different types of maintenance. Some devices may only need periodic cleaning (commodes and urinals). Other devices may require battery changes or servicing. The caregiver should be informed about the maintenance of any equipment used by the older adult in his or her care.

Call Bells and Personal Alarms

There are numerous call bells and personal alarms available for use by older adults. Most call bells have a push button of some type, although voice-activated devices are available. Some services make daily calls to older adults and notify family or emergency services if there is no answer. One type of personal alarm available for older adults has a base set and an alarm that is worn on a pendent around the neck or on a wrist strap. If the person falls or needs help, he or she presses the alarm. The alarm alerts a call center that sends assistance. There are alert alarm systems (movement sensors) that attach to the patient's clothes. These alarms are meant to prevent wandering. An alarm sounds if the person falls or gets out of the bed or chair. Movement sensors in stationary positions (such as by a doorway) sound an alarm if a patient walks or moves past the sensor. Door alarms sound when a patient tries opens a door.

Medication Dose Boxes

Medication dose boxes can improve medication compliance and ensure that the correct dose of medication is taken. Older adults may have difficulty opening medicine bottles, may forget if they have taken medication, and may skip a dose or take a double dose. If the adult is taking multiple medications, the issue becomes more confusing. Most medication dose boxes can be filled with a week's worth of medications. Some boxes are harder to open than others, so the patient may have to try several types of boxes. Even patients able to manage their own medications often prefer the timesaving measure of preparing all medications for the week at one time. Some dose boxes will accommodate medications taken three to four times daily, but the day and time should be clearly marked on the individual cell. For people who have trouble remembering to take medications, there are a number of helpful electronic devices that can be programmed to give a reminder. There are dose boxes that beep and watches that signal time to take medications. Pharmacies will put easy-opening lids on pill bottles on request and some pharmacies, such as Target, will color-code bottles for different family members.

Patient Current and Historical Functional Abilities

Functional abilities should be assessed while the adult is engaged in active behaviors. The adult should be asked to demonstrate the ability to sit, stand, get on and off of the toilet, walk, bend down, listen, read, answer questions, and remove shoes, shirt, or jacket and put them on again. Ideally, this should be in the home environment, but this is not always possible. Careful questioning by the nurse about distances and type of facilities in the home environment can help with approximating the type of activities required. The adult being assessed can walk up and down a hallway, for example, to approximate walking from the car to the front door. A careful history of functional ability can pinpoint the timing of any changes. Again, specific questioning should be used. For example, the nurse could ask, "When did you begin to use a cane?" or "How old were you when you stopped using the tub?"

Psychological, Social and Sensory Functioning

Functional status assessment concerns the ability to perform self-care and self-maintenance and to engage in physical activities. However, other factors may interfere with normal functioning. Tests of psychological function assess anxiety, worry, grief, and depression. Those with depression may be at increased risk of physical disability or may neglect self-care. Tests of social function assess support from family or friends, the need for a caregiver, financial resources, mistreatment or abuse, the ability to drive, and the presence of advance directives. Tests of sensory function assess the health of the sensory systems. These tests look for signs and symptoms of cataracts, glaucoma, myopia, presbyopia, astigmatism, macular degeneration, or eye disorders that make it difficult for people to read medication labels or do self-care. It should be determined if the adult needs audio materials or enlarged print. Hearing is evaluated in both ears for hearing deficits and high- and low-frequency hearing loss as well as waxy buildup in the ear canals.

Pneumococcal 23-Valent Polysaccharide Vaccine (PPV-23).

The pneumococcal 23-valent polysaccharide vaccine (PPV-23) (Pneumovax and Pnu-Immune) protects against 23 types of pneumococcal bacteria. Pneumococcal vaccine is now routinely administered to children. This practice has reduced the overall incidence of infection in both children and older adults. The vaccine is given to adults 65 years of age and over. The vaccine is also administered to individuals with chronic disease (sickle cell anemia, asplenia, Hodgkin's disease, chronic obstructive pulmonary disease [COPD], human immunodeficiency virus/acquired immune deficiency syndrome [HIV/AIDS], cardiopulmonary and liver disease, and diabetes) because they are at increased risk. Only one dose of the vaccine is usually required, although a second dose may be advised for individuals with some diseases (such as cancer) or those who have had organ/bone marrow transplantations. Revaccination is recommended for individuals older than age 65 if the first vaccination was administered five years or more previously and the patient was younger than 65 years of age at the time. Studies have indicated that this vaccine protects against pneumococcal bacteremia in older adults but is less successful in protecting against pneumonia, the primary form of pneumococcal infection.

Vaccines

Influenza Vaccine

A different influenza (flu) vaccine is formulated each year. Administration begins in September, prior to flu season. There are two types of flu vaccine: trivalent inactivated influenza vaccine (TIV) and live attenuated influenza vaccine (LAIV). TIV (injectable) is administered to those older than six months old, including older people who are healthy or have chronic medical conditions. LAIV is a nasal spray for use in those 2 to 49 years of age. The LAIV vaccine is not administered to pregnant women or older adults. Vaccination is recommended for people older than 50, people at high risk of contracting the flu (such as health-care providers), and caregivers (such as babysitters and grandparents) of children under six months of age. The flu vaccine is contraindicated for individuals with allergies to eggs, a history of reaction to the flu vaccine, and a history of Guillain-Barré syndrome. The vaccine should not be administered to those who received a previous vaccination within the last six weeks. Adverse effects include infection with local inflammation, fever, and aching.

Herpes Zoster Vaccine

Individuals who have had chicken pox as children or adults retain the varicella zoster virus in the nerve cells. The virus can become active in adulthood and cause herpes zoster (shingles). Herpes zoster occurs most commonly in those older than 50 years of age with chronic medical conditions and those who are immune-compromised. Since 2006, the herpes zoster vaccine has been recommended for individuals 60 years of age and older. A single dose of the vaccine is needed. Studies indicate that the herpes zoster vaccine prevents about 50 percent of herpes zoster cases and decreases the severity of the condition in those who still develop the disease. The vaccine is contraindicated for individuals with allergies to gelatin or neomycin and individuals who are immune-compromised due to human immunodeficiency virus/acquired immune deficiency syndrome (HIV/AIDS), chemotherapy, radiation, steroid use, history of leukemia or lymphoma, and active tuberculosis. Adverse reactions are rare and include allergic response, local inflammation, and headache.

Hepatitis B Immunizations

Hepatitis B can cause serious liver disease leading to liver cancer. It is transmitted through blood and body fluids; therefore, hepatitis B immunization is now recommended for all newborns, those under 18 years of age, and individuals in high-risk groups who are older than 18 years of age (drug users, men having sex with men, those with multiple sex partners, partners of those with hepatitis B virus, and health-care workers). Older adults with end-stage renal disease (including those receiving

hemodialysis), chronic liver disease, or human immunodeficiency virus/acquired immune deficiency syndrome (HIV/AIDS) should receive the vaccine. The vaccination is also recommended for individuals traveling to international destinations where hepatitis B is a problem. Older adults in correctional facilities, drug-abuse treatment facilities, dialysis facilities, and nonresidential day care facilities for people with developmental disabilities should be vaccinated. Three injections of monovalent HepB are required to confer immunity. Adverse reactions include local irritation and fever. Individuals with severe allergies to baker's yeast may suffer reactions to the vaccine.

Hepatitis A Immunizations

Hepatitis A causes serious liver damage that can result in death. Hepatitis A is spread through the feces of a person who is infected. Individuals with the disease may contaminate food and water. Outbreaks have been traced to restaurants and kitchens in large facilities. A hepatitis A vaccine is now routinely administered to children. Older adults may receive the two-injection series if they are considered at risk. Individuals with certain lifestyles (males who have sex with other males or illegal drug users) and certain medical conditions (chronic liver disease and those receiving clotting factor concentrates) are considered at high risk. The vaccine is recommended for those traveling to areas in which the disease is endemic. The vaccine is also recommended if outbreaks of the disease occur. Adverse reactions are mild and include soreness, headache, anorexia, and malaise, although severe allergic reactions can occur as with all vaccines.

Infections

Nosocomial Infection

A nosocomial infection is defined by the National Nosocomial Infections Surveillance

(NNIS) as a localized or systemic hospital-acquired infection that was not present or (incubating) in the patient at the time he or she entered the hospital. The infection may be caused by a toxin or pathogen. In some cases, infection may be evident within the first 24 to 48 hours, but other infections may not be evident until after discharge from the hospital. This is because incubation times and resistance vary. An infection that occurs after discharge but is hospital acquired is also nosocomial. A nosocomial infection is identified by laboratory analyses and clinical symptoms. A diagnosis of infection by an attending physical or surgeon is also considered acceptable identification. Colonization that is not causing an inflammatory response or evidence of infection is not considered nosocomial for reporting purposes. The most common nosocomial infections are Staphylococcus aureus and methicillin-resistant Staphylococcus aureus (MRSA).

Methicillin-Resistant Staphylococcus Aureus (MRSA)

Methicillin-resistant Staphylococcus aureus (MRSA) is caused by a mutation in S. aureus that confers resistance to methicillin (amoxicillin), other beta lactamase-resistant penicillins, and cephalosporins. First identified in 1945, MRSA has become endemic in hospitals. It is the cause of surgical site and bloodstream infections and pneumonia. More than half of S. aureus infections are now classified as MRSA. The mortality rate of MRSA is 21 percent. MRSA often colonizes the skin, especially in the anterior nares, and can easily spread through contact with contaminated surfaces or contaminated hands. Community-acquired as well as hospital-acquired infections are of grave concern. Prompt diagnosis and treatment with vancomycin or other antibiotics are essential. Standard and contact precautions with use of gloves, gown, and masks should be instituted if deemed appropriate. Droplet precautions should be taken in cases of pneumonia. Patients with MRSA should be placed in a private room or cohort room. Routine surveillance of high-risk patients or those with a previous history of MRSA should be conducted.

Clostridium Difficile Infection

Clostridium difficile is an anaerobic gram-positive bacillus that produces endospores. It is commonly found in health-care facilities, such as hospitals. Intestinal flora (microorganisms) normally provide resistance to C. difficile, but if the flora are disrupted by antibiotic use (or sometimes chemotherapeutic agents) and the host is an asymptomatic carrier or has acquired the infection during or after treatment, then C. difficile can begin to overgrow. C. difficile produces a lethal cytotoxin called toxin B. It also produces an endotoxin with cytotoxic action (toxin A) that causes fluid to accumulate in the colon and causes severe damage to mucous membranes. C. difficile causes more cases of nosocomial diarrhea than any other microorganism. All antibiotics can cause C. difficile infections, but clindamycin and cephalosporins are most frequently implicated. Symptoms of C. difficile infection vary widely from mild diarrhea to lethal sepsis. C. difficile can cause diarrhea, colitis, pseudomembranous colitis, and megacolon. Infection may not be obvious for weeks after completion of treatment with antibiotics.

Epidemiology and Risk Factors for Development of VRE and MDRE

Vancomycin-resistant enterococci (VRE) and multidrug-resistant enterococci (MDRE) create serious problems for health-care facilities. VRE was first identified in the United States in 1989. By 2004, VRE was the cause of one-third of all the infections acquired in intensive care units related to the use of vancomycin. There are several phenotypes, but two types are most common in the United States: VanA (resistant to vancomycin and teicoplanin) and VanB (resistant to just vancomycin). VRE infections are treatable by other antibiotics, but MDRE infections are increasingly resistant to two or more antibiotics, including vancomycin. Restriction of vancomycin use alone has not proven successful in controlling the development of VRE or MDRE because other antibiotics, such as clindamycin, cephalosporin, aztreonam, ciprofloxacin, aminoglycoside, and metronidazole are implicated. Prior antibiotic use is present in almost all patients with MDRE. Other risk factors include prolonged hospitalization and intraabdominal surgery.

The incidence of VRE infections has increased greatly in both intensive care units and medical/surgical units. Approximately 25 percent of enterococci infections are now classified as VRE. Patients who are immunocompromised or severely ill are at increased risk. Also at increased risk are those admitted to intensive care units or hospitalized for lengthy periods. VRE is also associated with antibiotic use, including vancomycin, clindamycin, and ciprofloxacin. VRE can occur systemically or infect the urinary tract or surgical sites. Some people are colonized but have no symptoms. These individuals may pose a threat to others as the bacterium may survive on surfaces for up to six days. A number of precautions should be taken to prevent the spread of infection. Infected patients should be placed in isolation. All individuals entering the patient's room should use barrier precautions (gowns, gloves, and masks). All individuals must wash their hands thoroughly after contact with the patient. Dedicated equipment should be used to treat infected patients in order to reduce transmission. There should be a policy to limit vancomycin use. Isolation rooms should be cleaned thoroughly.

Organization·Network/ Health System

Cost-Effective Drugs

Drugs are one of the most expensive aspects of medical care for patients. Even individuals with insurance drug coverage or Medicare Part D may incur considerable costs, especially when non-generic drugs are involved. Drug representatives exert great pressure on physicians to prescribe new drugs, and patients are often influenced by direct-to-consumer advertising. However, the nurse can help the patient ensure that drugs are prescribed based on need. Additionally, the benefits of the drugs must justify their cost. It is the responsibility of the nurse to act in the best interests of the patient and to educate the patient about drugs. If a less expensive drug is as effective as a more expensive or newer drug, then the nurse and patient should request that the less expensive drug be prescribed. The nurse should educate people about the use of generic drugs as a cost-saving measure. In most cases, generic drugs are as effective as name brand drugs.

Even with insurance and Medicare, older adults may incur huge medical costs. If a patient requires nursing care at home or in a facility, the costs can range from $4,000 to more than $8,000 monthly. This quickly depletes savings. Medicare strictly limits hospital and extended care stay as well as home health care. When a patient is no longer improving, the patient's care is not paid for until he or she is eligible for hospice care. This can happen in the case of a terminal illness or Alzheimer's disease. There are also limitations on hospice care. Long-term care is not provided by Medicare or most insurance policies. There is insurance available for this purpose, but these policies are expensive. This leaves patients and families with financial burdens that they sometimes cannot pay. If savings are depleted (and the amount allowed varies from state to state), and the patient needs long-term care, state Medicaid programs may pay. However, there are few facilities willing to take Medicaid patients because the reimbursement rate is low.

Assisted Living Facilities

There are a wide range of options in assisted living facilities. There are choices ranging from residential care facilities that house two to three patients in a home setting to large facilities with dozens or even hundreds of patients. Typically, nurses are not on duty. Therefore, medical assistance is limited. Services usually offered include staff on duty 24 hours a day to provide assistance if needed, provision of meals (two to three meals daily), cleaning, activities, and transportation. Costs vary widely from $500 per month to $10,000 per month. The goal of assisted living is to allow the patient to remain as independent as his or her physical and cognitive abilities allow. Residents often have individual apartments. Assisted living is usually limited to individuals with mild to moderate functional impairment, but licensure varies somewhat from state to state. Facilities focusing on patients with Alzheimer's disease may face further requirements, such as provision of a safe environment that prevents patients from wandering away from the facility.

Residential Care Facilities

A residential care facility is a type of assisted living/group home. A typical residential care facility is a large home with two or more patients cared for by a person (often nonmedical) licensed by the state. Depending on the number of patients, nursing aides may be available to assist patients. Residents are assisted with activities of daily living, such as bathing and dressing, as required. Meals are cooked for the residents. The facilities have supervised activities for the residents. It is usually required that the residents be ambulatory, but this may vary according to the facility and state regulations. Residential care facilities do not usually provide medical care, so patients needing treatments (other than assistance with taking medications or minor treatments) are seen by home health agency nurses. Medicaid may provide funds to house older adults in residential care facilities, but the reimbursement rate is low. For this reason, finding a residential care facility that accepts Medicaid patients can be difficult. The cost for residential care ranges from $500 a month to thousands of dollars per month for luxury facilities.

Skilled Nursing Facilities

Skilled nursing facilities (SNF, nursing homes) are licensed by states to provide both medical care (medications and treatment) and personal care (such as bathing, dressing, meals, and activities). Patients with insurance or Medicare may be transferred to an SNF after acute care in hospital. The length of stay at an SNF usually ranges from a few days to six weeks, depending on the patient's condition and progress. SNFs usually provide physical therapy and occupational therapy. They may also provide respiratory therapy. The purpose of SNF care is to provide transitional care between the hospital and the home environment. In some cases, patients who require medical care and cannot be cared for at home may remain in the SNF until death. Although Medicare will not pay for this, long-term insurance will cover the cost. State Medicaid programs may pay if certain restrictions (income, condition, and age) are met. Some patients pay privately. Costs range from about $4,000 to $10,000 per month.

Home Health Agencies

Home health agencies provide intermittent care in the home or in assisted-living facilities. Home health-care workers may be nurses (assessment, medications, and treatment); social workers; speech pathologists; physical and occupational therapists; and certified nurse aides (personal care). Home health agencies may provide professionals to draw blood for lab tests and administer intravenous fluids. Home health care allows patients to be released earlier from acute hospitals and skilled nursing facilities. Home health care is more cost effective than inpatient care. Some insurance companies pay for home health care. Medicare will cover the cost under certain conditions. The patient must be homebound and in need of skilled care less than seven days per week or less than eight hours each day for a period of less than 21 days. Home health-care services may not exceed 28 to 35 hours per week, depending on the needs of the individual patient. Medicare pays a set amount for each episode of care (60-day period), depending on the health-care condition.

Adult Day Care

Adult day care programs provide respite for caregivers of older adults who require supervision. Programs vary widely in their scope. Some provide care for a few hours two or three times a week. Some programs provide care for 40 to 50 hours a week to allow caregivers to attend work. The cost of the programs varies widely. Some nonprofit organizations charge a minimal fee based on income. Other organizations charge up to $300 per week. In some cases, an older adult is placed in an adult day care program to provide socialization, but more often it is because he or she has physical and/or cognitive impairment and needs supervision. Day care programs usually provide meals and activities. Many programs are set up to provide a secure environment to deal with older adults with mild to moderate dementia. Many programs are not staffed by medical personnel, but others may include nurses on the staff.

Senior Centers

Senior centers provide services and recreational activities for older adults. Some senior centers offer day care programs, but services are generally intended for individuals who do not require supervision or assistance. Programs vary in the services they provide. Some senior centers are open a few hours a week for meetings and recreational activities (Bingo, cards, or dancing, for example). Other centers are open daily and offer programs (such as educational classes), meals (often at low cost), and recreational activities. Some senior centers provide transportation to and from the center, and some sponsor low-cost bus tours and vacation packages. Many communities have senior centers, and retirement communities often revolve around the activities provided by these centers. Senior centers sometimes provide low-cost legal assistance and help in filling out tax forms. Most centers provide information about senior services available in the community and may assist people in getting help they need.

Respite Care

Respite care is designed to serve the caregiver rather than the older adult. There are a number of forms of respite care. Hospice care allows an older adult to be admitted to a skilled nursing facility for up to five days. In other programs, a nurse aide may be assigned to stay with the patient for a few hours while the caregiver leaves the home. In some cases, the caregiver may be provided with money to hire help in the home. Most respite programs are intended to provide relief for those providing long-term care to individuals with chronic or terminal diseases or dementia (usually related to Alzheimer's disease). Caregivers can easily feel overwhelmed with the constant demands of providing care, especially if patients are active at normal sleeping times (as often occurs with Alzheimer's patients) or can never be left unattended for safety reasons.

Acute and Sub-Acute Care

Patients requiring acute care are usually treated in hospital where diagnostic procedures (such as magnetic resonance imaging [MRI], computed tomography [CT] scan, lab tests, and x-ray) can be readily performed. Hospitals also have the sophisticated equipment necessary to monitor patients. Patients admitted to acute care facilities are usually extremely ill, requiring eight to nine hours of skilled nursing care daily. Physicians and highly skilled nursing staff are available for patients around the clock. Sub-acute care provides a level of care between that of an acute hospital and a skilled nursing facility, although skilled nurses are available around the clock. Sub-acute care patients usually require four to six hours of skilled nursing care daily but may receive intensive therapy. Sub-acute care units may be contained within an acute hospital, but they may also exist as completely separate facilities. Most sub-acute care units do not offer monitoring or sophisticated diagnostic equipment, so patients treated in sub-acute units often have chronic (rather than acute) disorders, such as acquired immune deficiency syndrome (AIDS), head trauma, and neuromuscular diseases.

Rehabilitation Centers

Rehabilitation centers may be separate departments in acute, sub-acute, or skilled nursing facilities. Rehabilitation centers may exist as separate facilities and focus solely on rehabilitation and improving a patient's ability to function. The purpose of these centers is to help patients remain as independent as possible. There is a wide variety of rehabilitative programs, including stroke and brain injury programs, cardiac health programs, and physical therapy for those with bone or muscle injuries. For example, rehabilitative physical therapy may be used to help older adults strengthen muscles and improve mobility after a hip fracture. Comprehensive rehabilitation programs usually offer speech and occupational therapists. Depending on the medical issue of concern, individual patients may need only a few hours of outpatient care or months of inpatient care. Rehabilitative treatment is increasingly utilizing computerized technology to assist patients. Insurance, Medicare, and Medicaid usually cover the cost of rehabilitative care that is indicated to improve functionality or prevent further deterioration.

Home Meal Delivery Programs

Home meal delivery programs (such as Meals on Wheels) provide nutritious meals for homebound older adults. The programs usually deliver meals five to seven days a week. The programs are often staffed by volunteers. The cost of a meal is usually $2 to $4, but this varies by program. Most programs deliver one hot meal a day and may provide food for one or two other meals (such as a sandwich for dinner and cold cereal for breakfast the next day). Requirements and age restrictions vary. Some programs serve individuals 60 years of age and over, and others serve individuals 65 years of age and over. For people with temporary disabilities, there may be a limit on length of service. While some programs are intended for individuals with low incomes, other programs do not have income restrictions. Most programs provide little choice in menu but may offer low-fat, low-salt, or low-carbohydrate diets. Many home meal delivery programs have waiting lists because the need outpaces the available resources.

Evidence-Based Practice Guidelines

Evidence-based practice guidelines are commonly used for such things as standing medicine orders or antibiotic protocols. However, decisions are often made based on biased expert opinion or on studies that lack internal and/or external validity. Evidence-based practice guidelines should be

established in a systematic way. It's important that decisions be based on solid evidence and not personal belief. The establishment of evidence-based practice guidelines does not ensure that they will be followed. Some individuals will resist changing their practices, so consideration must be given to implementation. A policy must be developed as to whether the use of the guidelines is mandatory or voluntary. In addition, it must be decided to what degree individual practitioners can choose other options. Rigid guidelines may be counterproductive. In some cases, establishing guidelines may affect cost reimbursement from third-party payers.

Hospice Care

Hospice care is designed to care for terminally ill individuals within the last six months of life. This period may be extended by physician authorization every 60 days. Medicare patients are covered for hospice care. The patient must be eligible for Medicare Part A, and a physician must certify that the patient is terminal with a life expectancy of six months or less. The patient (or responsible relative) must agree that the patient will receive hospice care rather than regular Medicare. The goal of hospice care is to maintain the person in the home environment. The patient is provided with home health aides and homemakers; durable goods (such as dressings, adult diapers, and underpads); counseling; and social worker assistance. Hospice care aims to manage the patient's pain and keep him or her comfortable. Routine home care is intermittent and must comprise 80 percent of total care. In-home continuous care is available for short periods of time in crisis. Inpatient hospice may be used for four to five days for symptom management and/or a five-day respite period for caregivers.

Rehabilitative Care

Rehabilitative care is composed of a number of different services, including physical, occupational, speech, and respiratory therapy:

Physical therapy:
Exercises to strengthen muscles and increase or maintain mobility may involve active and passive exercises as well as computer-/machine-mediated exercises (such as use of a stationary bicycle). Physical therapy is often needed after injury to bones and/or muscles and after strokes.

Occupational therapy:
Patients are taught modifications to activities of daily living that allow them to be as independent as possible. For example, patients might be taught safe methods of bathing or cooking. Patients may be provided with assistive devices. Patients who have had a stroke often receive occupational therapy.

Speech therapy:
In speech therapy, patients are helped to improve their production and patterns of speech. In addition, speech therapy can help to improve swallowing. Speech therapy is often used to help stroke patients and individuals with neuromuscular diseases.

Respiratory therapy:
In respiratory therapy, patients are taught to manage respiratory limitations through paced-breathing/walking exercises. In addition, patients are taught diaphragmatic breathing to increase their ability to function with lung disease.

Palliative Care

The purpose of palliative care is to make the patient comfortable during a chronic or terminal illness. It does not provide curative treatment. Palliative care is meant to improve the quality of life and relieve suffering. It neither prolongs life nor hastens death. The goals of palliative care include the relief of pain and the relief of symptoms (such as nausea or shortness of breath). In addition, palliative care provides support for the patient, caregivers, and/or family. It ensures that patients and their families receive psychosocial and spiritual support. Palliative care may provide bereavement services. While palliative care is often given in conjunction with hospice care, palliative care should begin prior to hospice care, because many issues, such as pain management, must be addressed prior to the last six months of the patient's life.

Restorative Care/Supportive Care

Restorative care is usually provided after an individual has sustained an injury (fractured hip) or suffered an illness (stroke). Restorative care aims to return the patient to optimal functioning and prevent complications. Restorative care often involves physical and occupational therapy. However, the scope of restorative care is more comprehensive and includes encouraging the patient to be as independent as possible and to improve as much as possible. Restorative care includes activities to improve psychosocial adjustment and the patient's self-image. The patient is encouraged to strive for short, achievable goals (lift a leg or hold a cup, for example). In this way, the patient can see that he or she is making progress. This aids in building confidence. New goals are set as old goals are reached. The purpose of supportive care is to reduce problems, complications, and symptoms associated with treatment or disease. For example, a patient receiving chemotherapy may receive supportive care to relieve nausea and vomiting. Supportive care also includes psychosocial support to deal with personal/financial issues and spiritual support to provide comfort.

Critical Pathways

Critical pathways are plans that involve diagnosis, procedure, or condition-specific care. Critical pathways involve the services of individuals from numerous disciplines. Critical pathways outline the steps in a patient's care and the expected outcomes. The pathways outline goals in patient care and the sequence and time of interventions taken to achieve those goals. Critical pathways may be developed for physician care or nursing care. Increasingly, critical pathways are being used as a method to improve and standardize care and decrease hospital stays. There are two basic types of pathways: guidelines and integrated care plan/pathways. Guidelines outline patient care. Documentation is not required to demonstrate that guidelines have been followed. The pathway may be in the form of a flow sheet, with different paths to follow depending on the patient's outcomes.

An integrated care plan/pathway must be followed. Documentation with dates and signatures is necessary to show that the steps have been carried out and to indicate specific outcomes. Pathways should be based on best practices. Their effectiveness should be monitored and evaluated to determine if modifications are needed.

Case Management

The gerontological nurse is often the person best suited to handle case management for older adults. This is particularly true for older adults who do not have family or caregivers available to assist them. Case management is used within acute, sub-acute, and skilled nursing facilities. The case manager chairs the interdisciplinary team responsible for the treatment of the patient and ensures that the needs of the patient are communicated to all members of the team. The case manager also ensures that all team members are focused on the same goal. As the patient moves back into the community, the case manager provides aid to the patient in securing any necessary social support services (such as home health care, transportation, and Meals on Wheels). The gerontological nurse acting as case manager supervises and manages all aspects of care to ensure continuity of care.

Plan of Care

The plan of care is developed from information gained from the patient interview, history, physical exam, and medical records. Once a problem list is generated, the nurse must review and prioritize the problems on the list and determine patient goals. The goals depend on the type and severity of the problem. Goals should be specifically related to the problem, measurable by some method, and attainable. Some problems (such as cardiac arrhythmias) can be resolved with treatment, so the goal will be the resolution of the problem. Other problems (such as chronic conditions) probably won't resolve, so the goal will be preventing deterioration or further complications. Some problems (terminal cancer) cannot be resolved, and deterioration of the patient's condition is inevitable, so the goal will be palliation and ensuring the patient's comfort.

The AACN Synergy Model

The AACN synergy model is based on three levels of quality outcomes: patient, nurse, and system. The six general indicators of quality outcomes derived from the patient, nurse, and system are as follows:
- Satisfaction of patient and family
- Rate of adverse incidents
- Rate of complications
- Adherence to discharge plans
- Mortality rate
- Length of stay in hospital.

Patient outcomes include functional change, behavioral change, trust, ratings, satisfaction, comfort, and quality of life. Nurse outcomes include physiological changes, the presence or absence of complications, and the extent to which care or treatment objectives were attained. System outcomes include recidivism, costs, and resource utilization.

Risk Stratification and Outcomes

<u>Risk stratification is a statistical process used to adjust for confounding differences in risk factors.</u> Confounding factors are those that confuse the data outcomes. For example, different populations, different ages, or different genders cannot be directly compared due to known and unknown differences between the groups. For example, if there are two physicians—one with primarily high-risk patients and the other with primarily low-risk patients—the same rate of infection (by raw data) would suggest that the infection risks are equal for both physicians' patients. However, high-risk patients are much more prone to infection, so in this case, risk stratification would demonstrate that the low-risk patients had a much higher risk of infection, relatively speaking. Risk stratification is also used to predict outcomes of surgery by accounting for various risk factors (including ASO score, age, and medical conditions). Risk stratification is an important element of data/outcome analysis.

Interpretation of Outcome Data

Outcome data is used to guide performance improvement activities. Outcome data provides evidence of how well a process works but does not supply the reason; therefore, outcome data must be evaluated accordingly. When outcome data is used for process improvement, there are certain problems that must be considered. First, outcome data does not provide sufficient risk stratification for complete validity. Second, it is difficult to accurately attribute the outcome data to any one step in a process without further study. For example, if outcome data shows a decline in deaths in an emergency department that recently changed trauma

procedures but doesn't account for the fact that a gang task force has successfully decreased drive-by shootings and killings by 70 percent, it might be assumed that changes in the emergency department altered the outcome data. In fact, if the data was adjusted for these external factors, the death rate may have increased.

Types of Outcome Data

There are different categories of outcome data, and some categories may overlap. When considering outcome data, the focus may be on the process or the outcome data itself. The team analyzing the data should clarify the purpose of reviewing the data and should understand how process and outcome data interrelate.

- Clinical: This category includes symptoms, diagnoses, staging of disease, and indicators of patient health.
- Physiological: This category includes measures of physical abnormalities, loss of function, and activities of daily living.
- Psychosocial: This category includes feelings, perceptions, beliefs, functional impairment, and role performance.
- Integrative: This category includes measures of mortality, longevity, and cost-effectiveness.
- Perception: This category includes customer perceptions, evaluations, and satisfaction.
- Organization wide clinical: This category includes readmissions, adverse reactions, and deaths.

Support Systems

Support systems can provide physical and emotional support for older adults. They can make a huge difference in the life of an older adult. People without adequate support systems may turn to health-care providers to fill this need. Support system types include formal, semiformal, and informal. Formal support systems are usually regulated by laws or statutes and provide social (social workers), financial (Social Security), and medical (Medicare, Medicaid) support based on legal requirements (such as age or income). Semiformal support systems include organizations or agencies that provide support in the way of goods or services to older adults and include senior centers, religious organizations, and charitable organizations. Informal support systems develop out of the social network of the older adult and may include family and friends. Only those who actually provide assistance in some way are part of the support system. Many adults have family and friends who are not willing or available to assist. These individuals do not form part of the support system.

Issues of Cultural Diversity

Issues of cultural diversity must always be addressed in the plan of care. It is not valid to assume that all members of an ethnic or cultural group have the same attitudes and opinions. However, basic cultural guidelines should be available to staff, addressing issues such as eye contact, proximity, and gestures. The nurse should take the time to observe family dynamics and determine if language barriers exist. If necessary, the nurse should arrange for translators to ensure that communication is adequate. In patriarchal cultures, such as the Mexican culture, the eldest male may speak for the patient. In some Muslim cultures, females will resist care by males. The attitudes and beliefs of the patient in relation to care and treatment must be understood, accepted, and respected. In some cases, the plan of care must include the use of healers. The plan of care must also ensure that cultural traditions are respected.

Handling Prejudice

Prejudice, unfortunately, is present in the health-care setting and may be exhibited by staff and patients. Prejudice may relate to racism, sexism, ageism, or sexual orientation. Any type of prejudicial (racist or otherwise) or culturally insensitive comments from staff should be reported to management, so they can be discussed. People may make remarks without realizing the effect of their words, so increasing awareness is important. Dealing with patients who make negative comments can be more difficult. This is especially true if the patient has dementia. People with dementia may make statements that they would not have made prior to their illness. These comments may not accurately reflect the person who existed prior to the cognitive impairment. However, people who were prejudiced before may become even more prejudiced. The patient should be told directly (often by a manager or supervisor) that the statements are inappropriate. Other strategies include distracting or redirecting the patient and trying to determine what prompted the remarks (for example, confusion, anxiety, or fear).

Environmental Safety

Environmental safety factors should be assessed within the adult's actual environment if at all possible. If this is not possible, careful questioning of the patient can elicit the necessary information. The nurse can draw diagrams and approximate floor plans with the patient's help. The patient can be asked to make drawings if he or she is capable. This process can help point out modifications that need to be made. Family members may also assist with the assessment, providing useful information. Some patients, especially the elderly, may be reluctant to admit that the home is cluttered or that they are unable to maintain the home environment in a sanitary condition. Brochures and handouts about home safety and assistive devices should be provided to the patient. In addition, contact names and numbers for equipment needed in the home should be supplied to the patient. A checklist should be compiled of all necessary changes or additions with specific details, such as "Install 18-inch grab bar across from toilet." In some cases, a social worker or occupational therapist should visit the patient.

Medical Record Review Processes

There are a number of different types medical record review processes, and many reviews are mandated by regulations and accreditation. Types of medical review processes include prospective, concurrent, retrospective, and focused.

- Prospective: This category includes all those steps taken before an event, such as assessing need before care is given, checking credentials before hiring, determining ability to pay prior to doing elective procedures, and gaining preauthorization from insurance companies.
- Concurrent: This category includes ongoing assessment while the patient is receiving care, verification of medical necessity for continued treatment, and appropriate use of resources. Concurrent review may include medical records, observations of care, incident reports, and special case studies.
- Retrospective: This review is done after care has been provided and provides a full picture of the continuum of care and its effectiveness. A retrospective review may look at the medical records and the results of prospective and concurrent reviews.
- Focused: This category includes reviews done for specific predetermined reasons, such as a specific diagnosis, procedure, or process. Criteria for case selection must be outlined.

Patient Flow Management

Patient flow management is a method of tracking patients. This technique assesses the practices of the organization that influence the quality of patient care. Patient flow management assesses the way the patient flows through the system from triage to treatment. The process includes evaluating methods of routing patients through the various services. Departments are often interdependent. Organizationwide utilization management allows the evaluation and integration of information and services. For example, admissions may depend on discharges, which may depend on completion of imaging or laboratory studies, which, in turn, may depend on transmission of orders and transportation of patients. Patient flow can be improved by determining what aspects of the patient flow process are not working effectively and making changes in these areas.

Quality Improvement: A Systematic Approach

The development of performance improvement actions plans usually begins with prioritizing problems after an initial period of monitoring and assessment. Teams should be assembled. Individual team members should be selected based on their knowledge of the problems and process and their commitment to improvement. There are a number of steps that should be taken. Systematic approaches should be taken to identify problems, conduct root cause analysis, and identify feasible changes in process. An action plan should be developed that outlines the expected outcomes of the change in process, chain of responsibility, time line, and methods of evaluation. A pilot test should be conducted. The data from the pilot test should be analyzed. Modifications to the change in process should be made if necessary after the pilot test. If necessary, further pilot tests should be conducted. The plan should be adopted by individuals, departments, and leadership.

Root Cause Analysis

Root cause analysis (RCA) is a retrospective attempt to determine the cause of an event. The event studied is often a sentinel event, such as an unexpected patient death or a cluster of infections. Root cause analysis involves interviews, observations, and review of medical records. The professional conducting the root cause analysis (RCA) traces essentially every step in hospitalization and care, including every treatment, every medication, and every contact. The RCA focuses on systems and processes rather than individuals. The investigation may uncover one root cause of the event or a number of causes. The RCA also must include a thorough review of the literature to ensure that any changes in the process resulting from the RCA are based on current best practices. Plans without RCA may not be productive. For example, if operative infections were caused by contaminated air, process improvement plans to increase disinfection of the operating room surfaces would not be effective.

Quality Improvement: Prevent Problem Recurrence

Problem solving in any medical context involves developing a hypothesis and then testing the hypothesis through the assessment of data. There are steps that should be taken to prevent the recurrence of a problem:

- Step 1 is to define the issue. Talk with the patient or family and staff to determine the nature of the problem. For example, the problem may have arisen due to a failure in communication or due to other issues, such as culture or religion.
- Step 2 is the collection of data. This may involve interviewing additional staff or reviewing documentation to gain a variety of perspectives.
- Step 3 is the identification of important concepts. It should be determined if there are issues related to values or beliefs.
- Step 4 involves considering the reasons for actions. The motivation and intentions of all parties should be ascertained to determine the reason for the problem.
- Step 5 is making a decision. A decision on how to prevent a recurrence of a problem should be based on advocacy and moral agency.

Quality Improvement: Outcome Measures

An outcome measure is used to determine the success or failure of a process. Both short-term and long-term outcomes are important in quality improvement. Short-term outcomes are directly related to the process. Based on the outcomes, the process can be modified if necessary. Long-term outcomes, however, often relate more to general quality of care and patient satisfaction and may be used retrospectively to evaluate the process or plan for future care. Outcomes serve as an indicator that a process is effective or ineffective. Planners should focus on identifying three types of outcome measures: 1) clinical (determines if there are positive results from clinical interventions); 2) customer functioning (includes indicators of ability to perform); and 3) customer satisfaction (includes meeting expectations and needs).

Strategies of Leadership: Independent Approach

Charismatic
A charismatic leader depends on personal charisma to influence people. This type of leader is often very persuasive but may recruit personal followers and relate to one group rather than the organization at large, thus limiting effectiveness.

Bureaucratic

A bureaucratic leader follows organization rules to the letter and expects everyone else to do the same. This type of leader is most effective in situations involving the handling of cash or dangerous work environments. The bureaucratic leader may command respect but may not be open to change.

Autocratic

An autocratic leader makes decisions independently and strictly enforces the rules. However, team members often feel left out of the process and may not be supportive. This type of leader is most effective in crisis situations, but may have difficulty gaining the confidence and commitment of staff.

Consultative

A consultative leader presents a decision and welcomes input and questions, although decisions rarely change. This type of leadership is most effective when gaining the support of staff is critical to the success of proposed changes.

Strategies of Leadership: Team Approach

Participatory

A participatory leader presents a preliminary decision to his or her staff and then makes a final decision based on input from staff members. This type of leadership is time consuming and may result in compromises that are not necessarily satisfactory to management or staff. However, this process is motivating for staff members because it makes them feel that their expertise is valued.

Democratic

A democratic leader presents a problem and asks staff members to come up with a solution, although the leader usually makes the final decision. This type of leadership may delay decision making, but staff members are often more committed to the solutions because of their input.

Laissez-faire

A laissez-faire leader exerts little direct control over staff members. Staff members make decisions with little interference. This may be effective leadership if the staff members are highly skilled and work well independently, but in many cases this type of leadership is the product of poor management skills, and little is accomplished because of lack of leadership.

Collaboration within the Nursing Profession

Nurses must learn the skill of collaboration in order to advance the profession of nursing. Nurses must take an active role in gathering data for evidence-based practice to support the profession's role in health care. Nurses must share their knowledge with other nurses and health professionals in order to plan staffing levels and to provide optimal care to patients. Adequate staffing has consistently been shown to reduce adverse patient outcomes, but there is a well-documented shortage of nurses in the United States; more than half of current RNs work outside the hospital. Increased patient loads not only increase adverse outcomes but also increase job dissatisfaction and burnout. In order to manage the challenges facing nursing, nurses must develop skills needed for collaboration. Nurses must be willing to compromise. They must be able to communicate clearly. Nurses must be able to identify specific challenges and problems and must be able to focus on the task at hand. Finally, nurses must be able to work collaboratively as part of a team.

Collaboration between the Nurse and Patient/Family

The collaboration between the nurse and the patient and or the patient's is extremely important but is often overlooked. Nurses and health-care providers must always remember that the point of collaborating is to improve patient care. This means that the patient and patient's family must remain central to all planning. Including the patient and his or her family in planning takes time initially but is very valuable. The patient and his or her family can provide information that facilitates planning and the expenditure of resources. Including the patient and family in planning can save money in the long run. Families, and even young children, often want to participate in care and planning and feel validated. This creates a more positive attitude toward the medical system.

Importance of Communication Skills

Collaboration requires a number of communication skills that differ from those involved in communication between nurse and patient. Collaboration requires the nurse to be assertive, but nonthreatening. The nurse must express her opinions honestly, clearly, and with confidence. The nurse must learn to make casual conversation. Establishing a personal connection can help in the collaboration process. This type of relationship can be established before meetings, during breaks, and after meetings. To collaborate effectively, the nurse must be competent in public speaking. The nurse must be able to present his or her ideas to groups of people. Public speaking is a skill that must be practiced. Collaboration also requires communicating in writing. The nurse must be able to communicate clearly, using grammatically correct language.

Delegation of Tasks

One major responsibility in the leadership and management of a performance improvement team is effective delegation. The purpose of forming a team is to share the workload. Leaders cannot perform effectively if they take on too much of the workload. Additionally, failure to delegate shows an inherent distrust in team members. The leader is ultimately responsible for the delegated work. Mentoring, monitoring, and providing feedback and intervention are necessary components of leadership. Delegation includes the following:

- Assessing the skills and availability of the team members, determining if a task is suitable for an individual
- Assigning tasks with a time line
- Ensuring that the tasks are completed properly and on time by monitoring progress but not micromanaging
- Reviewing the final results and recording outcomes.

The Five Rights of Delegation

Prior to delegating tasks, the nurse should assess the needs of the patient and determine the tasks that need to be completed. The nurse must ensure that he or she can remain accountable. The nurse must be able to supervise those carrying out the tasks and evaluate effective completion. The five rights of delegation include the following:

- Right task: The nurse should determine an appropriate task to delegate.
- Right circumstance: The nurse must consider the setting, resources, time factors, safety factors, and all other relevant information to determine the appropriateness of delegation.
- Right person: The nurse has the responsibility of choosing the right person (by virtue of education/skills) to perform a task for a specific patient.
- Right direction: The nurse must provide a clear description of the task and its purpose and expected outcomes.
- Right supervision: The nurse must be able to supervise and intervene as needed and evaluate the performance of the task.

Advocacy and Moral Agency

Advocacy is defined as working in the best interests of the patient and assisting patients to gain access to appropriate resources. The nurse must advocate for the patient even if there is a conflict with the nurse's personal values. Moral agency is defined as the recognition of the need to take action to influence the outcome of a conflict or decision.

There are three levels of advocacy/moral agency:

- Level 1: This nurse works on behalf of the patient. He or she is aware of patient's rights and ethical conflicts and advocates for the patient when it is consistent with the nurse's personal values.
- Level 2: This nurse advocates for the patient and family, incorporates the patient's values into the care plan even when they differ from the nurse's, and uses internal resources to assist the patient and his or her family with complex decisions.
- Level 3: This nurse advocates for the patient and family despite differences in values and is able to employ both internal and external resources to help empower the patient and/or family to make decisions.

The Vision Statement versus The Mission Statement

A Vision Statement is a description of what the organization intends to become. The vision statement outlines the commitment being made by the organization. It should include future goals rather than focusing on what has already been achieved; it is usually stated in one sentence or a short paragraph.

The Mission Statement of an organization usually reflects the current status of the organization and describes, in broad terms, the purpose of the organization and its role in the community. It should be developed in response to data and program analysis. The mission statement should be written with input from all members of the organization, and it should identify the organization or program, state its function, and outline the purpose and strategy of the program.

Organizational Policies, Procedures and Working Standards

Changes in policies, procedures, or working standards are common and staff should be educated about changes related to processes. Change should be communicated to staff in an effective and timely manner.

Policies are usually changed after a period of discussion and review by administration and staff, so all staff members should be made aware of policies under discussion. Preliminary information should be disseminated to staff members regarding the issue under consideration during meetings or through printed notices.

Procedures may be changed to increase efficiency or improve patient safety. Changes in procedures are often instituted as a result of surveillance and outcomes data. Procedure changes are best communicated in workshops with demonstrations. Handouts should be available as well.

Working standards are often changed because of regulatory or accrediting requirements. These changes may be required by regulatory agencies. Information on changes in working standards should be covered extensively so that the implications are clearly understood.

Regulatory Guidelines

The Health Insurance Portability and Accountability Act (HIPAA) addresses the rights of the individual regarding the privacy of health information. The nurse must not release any information or documentation about a patient's condition or treatment without the patient's consent. The patient has the right to determine who has access to personal information. Personal information about the patient is considered protected health information (PHI) and includes any identifying or personal information about the patient (such as health history, condition, or

- 122 -

treatments). Personal information includes documentation in any form, including electronic, verbal, or written. Personal information can be shared with a spouse, legal guardians, and those with durable power of attorney for the patient. Individuals involved in care of the patient, such as physicians, are also allowed access to personal information without a specific release. However, to ensure that he or she has no objections, the patient should always be consulted if personal information is to be discussed while others are present. Failure to comply with HIPAA regulations can make a nurse liable for legal action.

Patient Self-determination

In accordance with Federal and state laws, individuals have the right to self-determination in health care. This includes the right to make decisions about end-of-life care through <u>advance directives</u> (living wills). The patient also has the right to assign a surrogate person to make decisions through a durable power of attorney. Nurses should routinely ask patients about an advanced directive because the patient may present at a health-care organization without the document. Patients who have a Do-Not-Resuscitate (DNR) order should not receive resuscitative treatments for terminal illness or conditions in which meaningful recovery cannot occur. Patients and families of those with terminal illnesses should be questioned as to whether the patients are hospice patients. For those with DNR requests or in the case of withdrawal of life support, staff should provide palliative rather than curative measures. Palliative measures include pain control and/or oxygen, and emotional support. Religious traditions and beliefs about death should be treated with respect.

Education

Learning Styles

There are several preferred learning styles. Not everyone is aware of the style that suits them best. A range of teaching materials that relates to all three learning preferences (visual, auditory, and kinesthetic) should be available. Part of teaching involves choosing the right approach based on observation and feedback. Often, presenting learners with different options gives a clue to their preferred learning style. Some people have a combined learning style. Visual learners learn best by seeing and reading. The teacher should provide written directions, picture guides, or demonstrate procedures. The teacher should use charts, diagrams, photos, and videos. Auditory learners learn best by listening and talking. The teacher should explain procedures while demonstrating and having the learner repeat the instructions. The teacher should plan extra time to discuss and answer questions. Educational videos should be provided. *Kinesthetic* learners learn best by handling, doing, and practicing. The teacher should provide hands-on experience throughout the lesson. The teacher should encourage the handling of supplies and equipment. The learner should be allowed to demonstrate the lesson.

Characteristics of Adult Learners

Adult learners have a variety of life and/or employment experiences. Learning characteristics depend, in large part, on the personality of the learner. Learners may be practical and goal-oriented, self-directed, knowledgeable, relevancy-oriented, or motivated. Learners may be a combination of these categories.

Practical and goal-oriented individuals should be provided with overviews or summaries and examples. The teacher should conduct collaborative discussions with problem-solving exercises.

Self-directed individuals like to be actively involvement in the learning process. The teacher should allow different options toward achieving the goal. The learner should be given responsibility.

Knowledgeable learners should be shown respect for their life experiences and/or education. The teacher should validate their knowledge and ask for feedback. New material should be related to information with which they are familiar.

Relevancy-oriented learners like to know how the information to be learned relates to the problem. The teacher should explain how the information learned will be applied. Objectives should be clearly identified.

Motivated learners like a goal to work towards. They should be provided with certificates of achievement or some type of recognition for achievement.

One-On-One versus Group Instruction for Patient/Family Education

One-on-one instruction is the most costly type of instruction for an institution to conduct because it is time intensive. However, it allows the patient and family more time to interact with the nurse instructor and allows them to have more control over the process. The patient and family can ask questions or ask the instructor to repeat explanations or demonstrations. One-on-one instruction is especially valuable when patients and families must learn particular skills, such as managing dialysis. It is also a good method if confidentiality is important.

Group instruction is less costly than one-on-one instruction because the needs of a number of people can be met at the same time. Group presentations are more structured and are usually scheduled for a particular time-limited period (an hour, for example). Therefore, patients and families have less control over the instruction process. Questioning by patients is usually more limited and may be done only at the end of the session. Group instruction allows patients and families with similar health problems to interact. Group instruction is especially useful for general instruction, such as managing diet.

Behavior Modification and Compliance Rate

Education, like all interventions, must be evaluated for effectiveness. The following are two determinants of effectiveness: behavior modification and compliance rates.

Behavior modification involves the identification of behavior that needs to be changed and the institution of interventions to modify that behavior. A variety of techniques are used in behavioral modification, including demonstrations of appropriate behavior, reinforcement, and monitoring until new behavior is consistent. A gerontological nurse can carry out these techniques. Long-standing procedures and habits of behavior are particularly resistant to change.

Compliance rates are often determined by observation. The patient should be observed at frequent intervals. However, observation may involve patient self-reports. Outcome is another measure of compliance; the reduction of risk factors and improvement of patient health are good indications of compliance. Compliance rates are calculated by determining the number of events and procedures.

Learner Outcomes

The nurse should identify the educational outcomes of any educational experience. The outcomes should be conveyed to the learners from the very beginning so that they are aware of the expectations. The subject matter of the educational material and the learner outcomes should be directly related. There may be one outcome or a number of outcomes involved. A large task may be broken down into smaller tasks. For example, if the nurse is instructing a patient on preparing and giving insulin injections, then a learner outcome might be to accurately fill the syringe with the correct insulin dose. The assessment at the end of the educational experience determines if the outcomes were met. A survey of whether or not the learners felt that they had achieved the learner outcomes can give valuable feedback and guidance to the educator.

Professional Development

Continuing education is the education and training that are required to remain current in the nursing profession. Continuing education is an obligation of all nurses. Employers may require continuing education for continued employment. In some cases, employers may require that nurses take specific courses or types of courses. Continuing education requirements for renewal of an RN license (regardless of the type of program) are established by individual states and vary widely. Some states require no continuing education. Other states require a minimum number of units (one contact hour per unit). This often comes out to 20 to 30 units for each licensing period, which is typically every two years. Some states specify certain courses that must be taken for license renewal (end-of-life or human immunodeficiency virus/acquired immune deficiency syndrome [HIV/AIDS], for example). State boards of nursing must approve all providers of continuing education courses. This is to ensure that the courses meet minimum standards. Continuing education courses may be delivered in a traditional classroom setting, via the Internet, or through self-study materials.

Certification

Certification as a gerontological nurse specialist is evidence of expertise in the field. The American Nurses Credentialing Center provides certification for nurses with associate degrees (RN, certified) and bachelor's degrees (RN, board certified). To take the examination for certification, the nurse must meet the following basic requirements: two years' experience as an RN, 2,000 hours or more of clinical gerontological practice within the previous three years, and 30 units of continuing education in gerontological nursing.

Recertification requirements include current nursing license and fulfillment of at least two out of the following five categories of professional development:

- Continuing education: Seventy-five contact hours with more than 51 percent related to specialty.
- Academic credits: Five semester/six quarter units related to specialty.
- Presentations: Five different professional presentations related to specialty and not required by employment.
- Publication or research: An article in a peer-reviewed journal or book chapter or development of educational materials (such as DVDs, CDs, and Internet materials) related to specialty or performance as primary investigator for a research project related to specialty.
- Preceptorship: One hundred twenty or more hours of supervision of nursing students in a certification specialty.

*Note: Categories 1 to 4 may be counted twice by doubling their requirements

Professional Development: Credentials for Advanced Nursing

Clinical nurse specialists in gerontology, board certified (GCNS-BC), and gerontological nurse practitioners, board certified (GNP-BC), must have completed a minimum of a master's degree in nursing. There are specific requirements for the certification examination. Recertification requirements are similar to those for the gerontological nurse specialists RN-C and RN-BC.

Gerontological Nurse Practitioner:
A GNP-BC must have an active RN license and a master's degree or PhD. He or she must have completed 500 or more faculty-supervised clinical hours in a gerontological nurse practitioner program. The program must include courses in advanced health assessment, pharmacology, and pathophysiology as they relate to older adults. The nurse must have completed life-span education that includes health promotion and disease prevention. He or she must have acquired the skills to provide a differential diagnosis and manage diseases.

Clinical Nurse Specialist:
A GCNS-BC must have an active RN license and a master's degree or PhD. He or she must have completed 500 or more faculty-supervised clinical hours in the area of specialty. Course work must include advanced health assessment, pharmacology, and pathophysiology.

Research

Informed Consent

The patient or the patient's family must give informed consent for all treatment the patient receives or for any study in which the patient participates. The physician must give a thorough explanation of all procedures and treatment and the associated risks. Patients and/or their families should be apprised of all options and be allowed input on the treatments administered. Patients and/or their families should be made aware of all risks and any complications that might be life threatening or increase morbidity. The American Medical Association has established guidelines for informed consent. The patient and/or family must receive the following information:

- Explanation of diagnosis
- Nature and reason for treatment or procedure
- Risks and benefits of proposed treatment or procedure
- Alternative options (regardless of cost or insurance coverage)
- Risks and benefits of alternative options
- Risks and benefits of not having a treatment or procedure.

Human Subject Protection

The Food and Drug Administration's Code of Federal Regulations, title 21, volume 1, regulates the protection of human subjects. The regulations state that any researcher involving patients in research must obtain informed consent in language understandable to the patient or the patient's agent. The research must be explained to the patient. The patient must be informed about the purpose and the expected duration of the research. Any potential risks and benefits must be described. Possible alternative treatments must also be described. Any

compensation to be provided must be outlined. The extent of confidentiality should be clarified. Contact information should be provided in the event the patient/family has questions. The patient must be informed that participation is voluntary and that he or she can withdraw from participation at any time without penalty. Informed consent must be documented by a signed, written agreement.

Hypothesis and Hypothesis Testing

A hypothesis is preliminary statement devised to explain an observed phenomenon. Hypotheses are used in scientific research. A hypothesis must be testable. The scientific method involves the testing of a specific hypothesis. Scientific hypotheses are based on previous observations of a phenomenon or are extension of existing theories. The scientific method requires a hypothesis to be formulated. An experiment or study, which involves the gathering and analysis of data, is then designed to determine if the hypothesis is correct. The outcome of the experiment either supports the hypothesis or does not support the hypothesis. If the hypothesis is not supported, a new method of testing is devised or a new hypothesis is formulated.

Internal validity is concerned with the accuracy of the results of an experiment or study. If an experiment or study has internal validity, it demonstrates a cause and effect relationship between the variables that truly exists.

External validity is concerned with whether or not the results of an experiment or study are representative of the larger population.

Generalizability is concerned with whether or not the results of an experiment or study apply to other populations than the one studied.

Replication is concerned with whether the same results will be obtained if an experiment or study is repeated. The results of an experiment are considered to be sound if an experiment or study can be repeated and the same results are obtained.

Qualitative and Quantitative Data

Qualitative research involves subjective analysis. The property being studied cannot be enumerated. Qualitative data is a measure of the quality or character of the property in question. Qualitative data is classified as nominal or ordinal. Qualitative data may still be systematically analyzed. Patterns of responses are often organized into categories for analysis. Asking a person to describe his or her experience in a hospital involves collecting qualitative data.

Quantitative research measures the quantity or range of a property. This type of data is objective. Quantitative data can be expressed in numerical form. Quantitative data is obtained when the property in question can be measured. For example, measuring the difference in height between men and women involves collecting quantitative data.

Critical Reading Skills

Nurses should be able to use critical reading skills to evaluate material in the literature. The source of the material must be considered. Material published in the popular press may have little validity compared to material published in a refereed journal. The author's credentials should be taken into consideration. An author may or may not be an expert in the field of study in question. The thesis, which is the central claim of the research, should be clearly stated. The theoretical standpoint of the article should be examined. The methodology used should be assessed for soundness. The statistical evidence should be reviewed to determine if the results support the conclusions. The findings should be assessed for generalizability. The overall article should be assessed to determine if the information seems credible and useful and if it should be communicated to administration and/or staff.

Practice Test

Practice Questions

1. In assessing the aging client, it is important for the nurse to recognize?
    a. The client's ability to perform activities of daily living
    b. The financial status of the client
    c. The job that the client held prior to aging
    d. All components of well-being, including biological function, psychological function, and social function

2. Medications, slower mobility, lack of proper fluid intake, and poor diet can contribute to what common symptom in the elder population?
    a. Urinary incontinence
    b. Skin changes
    c. Mental changes
    d. Depression

3. The nurse assessing the older population needs to have a basic understanding of which of the following?
    a. The economic status of the area
    b. The difference between normal and abnormal for the older age group
    c. The signs of sexual dysfunction
    d. The signs of cardiac disease

4. Which statement would be most appropriate to ask when assessing an aging adult for cognitive function?
    a. What is today's date?
    b. Can you count to 10 for me?
    c. Have you noticed anything different about your memory or thinking in the past few months?
    d. Who is the president of the United States?

5. Which disease or ailment is often under diagnosed and undertreated in the aging population?
    a. Schizophrenia
    b. Depression
    c. Associative disorders
    d. Attention deficit disorder

6. Which statement demonstrates normal cognitive function for an aging adult?
    a. Occasional memory lapses
    b. Unable to recall the names of their children or siblings
    c. Unable to recall current address or phone number
    d. Unable to count to 10 or repeat a series of consecutive numbers

7. Dementia and depression are strongly related to?
   a. Clients over the age of 60
   b. Clients over the age of 65
   c. A decreased quality of life and functional deficits
   d. Past economic status and job performance

8. Which statement reflects the state of drug absorption in the geriatric patient?
   a. The rate of absorption is slowed
   b. The rate of absorption is faster due to thinning of mucosa
   c. The percent of the medication that is absorbed is decreased
   d. There is a decrease in gastric pH as we age

9. The absorption of medication in the geriatric client is most often affected by?
   a. A decrease in body fat
   b. An increase in serum albumin
   c. A decrease in body water and lean body weight
   d. An increase in body water

10. Which organ is responsible for drug metabolism and must be considered when prescribing medications for an older adult?
   a. Kidneys
   b. Pancreas
   c. Intestines
   d. Liver

11. An older adult on digoxin and furosemide is showing signs of toxicity. The gerontology nurse understands that?
   a. Digoxin and furosemide are excreted by the kidneys, and the doses may need to be decreased due to impaired kidney function
   b. Digoxin and furosemide are excreted through the intestinal tract, and dose changes would be ineffective
   c. An increase in fluid intake will fix the symptoms, and no change in dose is needed
   d. How a drug is excreted is not a consideration when dosing an older adult

12. Which statement is true regarding adverse drug reactions (ADRs) in older adults?
   a. The rate of ADRs in geriatric clients is seven times that of younger adults and poses serious health problems
   b. Older adults rarely have adverse reactions to prescribed medications because they are monitored
   c. Adverse reactions are minimal in older adults and require no intervention
   d. Only about 1% of older adults require hospitalization for ADRs

13. Which substance(s) show changes through aging by becoming less pliable and stiffer?
   a. Lipofuscin
   b. Collagen and elastin
   c. Epithelial tissue
   d. Cytoplasm

14. Which factor is NOT a normal part of aging and needs to be addressed to promote nutrition in the older adult client?
    a. Loss of teeth
    b. Increase in gastric pH
    c. Xerostomia or dry mouth
    d. Decline in basal metabolic rate

15. An 80-year-old female asks the nurse about over-the-counter vitamin supplements. The most appropriate advice would include:
    a. No vitamin supplements are needed with a balanced diet
    b. Any multivitamin will do
    c. Take only a calcium supplement
    d. Take a multivitamin for those over the age of 50, which should include the recommended vitamins for the aging adult

16. Which theories on aging were introduced in the early 1900s?
    a. Wear-and-tear theory and autointoxication theory
    b. Evolution theory
    c. Molecular theory
    d. Cellular theory

17. Systems theory includes which components about aging?
    a. Gene regulation ideas
    b. Mutation accumulation on aging
    c. Neuroendocrine and immunological ideas
    d. Free radical ideas

18. What is the most noticeable change in tissue as it ages?
    a. Decrease in lipids
    b. Increase in subcutaneous tissue
    c. Decrease in wrinkles
    d. Accumulation of pigmented material called lipofuscin

19. What is the most significant change in vital organs in the aging client?
    a. No change in organ tissue is noted
    b. The outer appearance of an organ changes, but the functional component does not change
    c. Organs show signs of decrease in function during the aging process
    d. The aging process speeds up the functional capacity of major organs

20. What benefit does evidence-based practice offer clients over the age of 60?
    a. No actual benefits have been noted when evidence-based practice is the model for geriatric care
    b. Evidence-based practice offers the client improved health care in all settings
    c. Evidence-based practice is only used as a model in acute care settings
    d. Minimal changes in geriatric care have arisen from the use of evidence-based practice models

21. What is the purpose of Rogers' diffusion of innovation model in relation to evidence-based practice (EBP)?
   a. There is no relation to EBP
   b. It offers an explanation of aging
   c. It is used to open communication around issues of implementing changes in practice when EBP research has shown that change would improve outcomes
   d. It is the model that contradicts the EBP theory

22. Which of the following statements defines who is appropriate for gerontological nursing care as stated by Orem (1991)?
   a. Orem (1991) refers to advanced pediatric nursing care
   b. Any aged client whose self-care demands exceed their ability to meet those demands is appropriate
   c. Orem (1991) refers to young adult nursing care in preparation for a healthy older adult life stage
   d. Any client who needs nursing care for whatever reason at any age is appropriate

23. Describe the order for the nursing process as practiced by the gerontological nurse.
   a. Diagnose, implement, evaluate
   b. assess, identify expected outcomes, implement, evaluate
   c. assess, diagnose along with the team, identify outcomes, plan, implement, evaluate
   d. assess, evaluate, plan, implement, and look at outcomes

24. Which choice best explains the practice setting for the gerontological nurse?
   a. In the home of the client
   b. Only in acute care settings
   c. Clinics and long-term care facilities
   d. Home of the client, acute care facilities, long-term care settings, and clinics or anywhere clients over the age of 65 seek health care and health education

25. A 70-year-old presents to the clinic stating that his family thinks he is losing his mind and they want to put him in a home. What would be the initial role of the gerontology nurse?
   a. Begin the process of finding a qualified nursing home
   b. Do a complete history, physical, and assessment
   c. Speak with the family about their concerns
   d. Make light of the subject until the nurse can evaluate the situation

26. Which item would not be a focus of a cognitive-perceptual pattern assessment for the older client?
   a. Cognition—Have you experienced any changes in your memory?
   b. Communication—Have you had any difficulty speaking or forming ideas?
   c. Financial—Have you had any financial hardships over the past several months?
   d. Orientation—Do you know what day, month, and year it is?

27. Which topic should NOT be omitted when assessing the aging client?
   a. Sexual history
   b. Cardiac history
   c. History of abuse
   d. All of the above

28. Which statement describes the importance of understanding nursing theory when practicing gerontology nursing?
   a. Understanding and using tested theories offer a framework on which to base nursing practice interventions
   b. Nursing theories are vague and do not offer substance in most health-care settings
   c. Theories are not proven ways on which to base nursing practice
   d. Theory helps identify major concepts in nursing practice and offers a framework for decision making

29. Kolcaba's (1994) theory of comfort supports which nursing practice standard?
   a. It supports transcultural nursing practice
   b. It supports basic nursing care, promoting the comfort of the patient
   c. It supports the importance of social support to buffer life's stresses
   d. It supports helping the patient to adapt to chronic illnesses

30. What is one important consideration when dealing with the older population when considering safety and medications?
   a. The older adult is at risk for falls, leading to an increase in morbidity and death
   b. A fractured arm is the highest risk for the older adult
   c. Depression is common in older adults and needs not be treated with medication
   d. Most older adults are not as fragile as was previously thought

31. The gerontological nurse may prescribe corticosteroids for all but which one of these conditions?
   a. Arthritis
   b. Hyperglycemia
   c. Allergic reactions
   d. Inflammatory states

32. An 80-year-old female decides on a do not resuscitate (DNR) status for herself after discussing her medical concerns with her physician. Which statement best describes the reasoning behind this decision?
   a. This is ethical reasoning based on self-determination and informed consent
   b. This is not a medical decision
   c. This discussion would be meaningless because the family members were not involved
   d. This is not an ethical decision

33. The nurse recognizes that cumulative changes in the skin of the elderly that are related to environmental factors are termed?
   a. Sunburned
   b. Photoaging
   c. No term exists to describe this
   d. Mole or blemish

34. The major portion of the dermis consists of what substance?
   a. Sebaceous glands
   b. Hair follicles
   c. Collagen
   d. Blood vessels and nerves

35. The cosmetic side of aging poses which effect on many older adults?
   a. The physical effect of sagging cheeks
   b. Psychological, affecting self-esteem and causing depression
   c. No notable effect
   d. No effect because older adults are mature enough to understand the aging process

36. Senile purpura significantly increases with age and is most related to?
   a. The aging process past the age of 60
   b. Related to increase in blood vessels
   c. Related to loss of subcutaneous fat and connective tissue
   d. Related to medications

37. The most common cause of death from skin cancer in the elderly is:
   a. Basal cell carcinoma
   b. Squamous cell carcinoma
   c. Malignant melanoma
   d. Actinic keratosis

38. The nurse understands that the goal for treatment of leg ulcers in the elderly client should be to?
   a. Relieve pain and swelling
   b. Relieve immobility
   c. Promote circulation
   d. Alleviate swelling, eliminate infection, and promote healing

39. Changes in bone and muscle in the aging population have the greatest effect on?
   a. Stature, posture, and function
   b. Appearance
   c. Immunity
   d. Pain tolerance

40. The nurse caring for the elderly population understands that movement slows with aging. This is most likely due to:
   a. Cognitive function
   b. Changes in musculoskeletal and nervous systems
   c. Laziness and a feeling that life is over
   d. A recent change in medical condition

41. The nurse recognizes that involuntary movements may appear in the elderly patient and be normal. These normal involuntary movements may present as which of the following?
   a. Seizures
   b. Tongue protrusions
   c. Resting tremors
   d. Eye twitches and spasms

42. The disease affecting adults over the ages of 55 to 60 where there is excessive resorption and deposition of bone is:
    a. Paget's disease
    b. Osteoporosis
    c. Wright's disease
    d. Scott's disease

43. A 69-year-old female presents with knee pain. The nurse hears a dry crackling or grating sound and the client feels the same sensation on exam. The nurse recognizes this as:
    a. Nothing abnormal for the age of the client
    b. Crepitation, the sound of osteoarthritis in the knee joint
    c. Osteoporosis and a softening of the knee joint
    d. Fluid-filled spaces in the knee joint

44. The nurse may recommend which of the following for the older client with mild arthritis?
    a. Complete bedrest
    b. Rest and ice for the joints affected
    c. A mild exercise program including walking
    d. No exercise will improve arthritis

45. A male elderly client on long-term auranofin therapy presents with oral ulcers and a pruritic rash and complaints of decreased urinary output. The nurse understands that:
    a. These symptoms can be the adverse effects of gold salt therapy
    b. These symptoms are unrelated to anything and need a major work-up for diagnosis
    c. These symptoms represent liver failure
    d. These symptoms are common when clients are treated for arthritis

46. The gerontological nurse understands that nonsteroidal anti-inflammatory drugs (NSAIDs) used for arthritis pain may cause?
    a. No side effects
    b. Liver failure in the first 24 hours
    c. Coagulation impairment and gastric irritation
    d. Fear or anxiety

47. The nurse is evaluating a 64-year-old male for coronary artery disease (CAD). Understanding that CAD is the leading cause of mortality, which risk factor would not be related to CAD?
    a. Hypertension
    b. Dyslipidemia
    c. Diabetes
    d. Sexual orientation

48. What is the single most cost-effective discovery made in the past 30 years that has influenced the prevention and treatment of cardiovascular events?
    a. The development of oral hypoglycemic drugs
    b. Recognizing the need to lower blood pressure in older adults
    c. Antismoking campaigns
    d. Zero tolerance for drug and alcohol abuse in older adults

49. The nurse evaluates a 70-year-old female who has been recording her blood pressures for the last few days. These pressures were 140/90, 146/90, 146/92, 138/88, and 150/89. The nurse recognizes this as the beginning of which stage of hypertension?
   a. Stage 2
   b. High normal blood pressures
   c. Stage 1
   d. Stage 3

50. The nurse is doing a follow-up clinic visit for a 75-year-old female post-cerebrovascular accident (CVA) of two months. The nurse should be prepared to discuss all of these possible complications except:
   a. Neurogenic bladder
   b. Depression
   c. Financial concerns
   d. Fecal incontinence

51. Which symptom is the most common with peripheral artery disease (PAD)?
   a. Intermittent claudication
   b. Warm extremities
   c. Pain unrelieved by rest
   d. Bounding pulses

52. The nurse is examining a 76-year-old female with the complaints of fatigue, ankle swelling, and mild shortness of breath over a three-week period. An appropriate nursing diagnosis might include:
   a. Decreased cardiac output related to altered contractility and elasticity of cardiac muscle
   b. Activity tolerances due to compensation of oxygen supply
   c. Increased cardiac output related to an aging heart muscle
   d. Decreased urinary output due to poor kidney perfusion

53. Factors that may further decrease lung function besides aging include all but:
   a. Smoking
   b. Obesity
   c. Immobility
   d. Exercise

54. Which choice would not be a nursing goal when managing chronic obstructive pulmonary disorder (COPD) in an older adult patient?
   a. Decreasing exercise
   b. Preventing and treating complications
   c. Reducing mortality risks
   d. Relieving symptoms

55. When caring for an older adult with pneumonia, the nurse recognizes all of the following are appropriate interventions except:
   a. Monitoring rate, rhythm, depth, and effort of respirations
   b. Auscultating breath sounds
   c. Monitoring blood sugars and reports BS higher than 145
   d. Monitoring for increased restlessness or anxiety indicating air hunger

56. Vertigo in the older adult is best described as:
   a. A vestibular disorder producing a rotational sensation
   b. A dysfunction of sensory signals
   c. A transient loss of consciousness
   d. A light-headed feeling

57. All statements are examples of nonpharmacological nursing interventions for a patient experiencing delirium but needing sleep except:
   a. Providing adequate sleep and awake times
   b. Encouraging ambulation
   c. Providing a night light to prevent fears
   d. Reducing noise levels during periods of sleep

58. Which statement best describes the procedure for assessing for the presence of Helicobacter pylori in the older adult patient?
   a. Colonoscopy
   b. Prescribing two weeks' worth of antibiotics, and then performing a colonoscopy
   c. Gastric biopsy, serum blood antibody studies, or stool assay exam
   d. Fecal occult blood exams

59. The nurse evaluating an elderly male client for urinary complaints understands that the major change in the prostate during the aging process is?
   a. Hyperplasia
   b. Renal stones causing obstructions
   c. Hypoplasia
   d. Impotence and embarrassment

60. Which statement best describes the nurse's understanding of normal expected sexual responses in aging female clients?
   a. No changes in sexual responses are noted with aging females
   b. Aging females experience a quicker arousal phase
   c. An aging female will most often experience a delayed arousal phase during intercourse
   d. An increase in vaginal secretions may be noted in the aging female

61. When assessing an aging client's genitourinary system, the gerontological nurse recognizes the importance of screening for:
   a. Drug addiction
   b. Bladder malignancy
   c. Diabetes
   d. Cognitive abilities

62. The gerontological nurse understands that the purpose for prescribing Ditropan is:
   a. An underactive kidney function
   b. Increasing contractions of the sphincter muscles
   c. Decreasing bladder muscle tone and aiding in urge incontinence
   d. Improving urogenital symptoms caused by vaginitis

63. Treatment approaches for an aging adult experiencing overflow incontinence may include all of the following except:
    a. Toilet schedule
    b. Positioning and the Crede maneuver
    c. Clean self-catheterizations
    d. Kegel exercises

64. Symptoms of hyperthyroid disease may include all of the following except:
    a. Heat intolerance
    b. Palpitations
    c. Tremors
    d. Diarrhea

65. The nurse recognizes the most common eye-related disease affecting the older adult is:
    a. Glaucoma
    b. Cataracts
    c. Near-sighted visual disturbances
    d. Far-sighted visual disturbances

66. The nurse should be aware that the percent of aging adults in a nursing home/long-term care setting experiencing sensory hearing loss is:
    a. 40%
    b. 60%
    c. 30%
    d. 70 to 80%

67. Which age-related psychological change is not the norm?
    a. An increased ability to multitask
    b. Lower scores on tests of creativity
    c. Thinking of death as a process rather than a moment in time
    d. Life satisfaction is related to well-being

68. Examples of health-care reimbursement or delivery modes include all of the following except:
    a. Medicaid
    b. Medicare
    c. Managed care, telemedicine, and case management
    d. Anthem for the elderly A/B

69. The program designed to supplement Social Security for those who do not qualify for Social Security or who are disabled is:
    a. OAA
    b. SSI
    c. Medicare
    d. Medicaid

70. The purpose of the Patient Self Determination Act is?
   a. To encourage patients to document their choices about life support and advance directives
   b. To help older adults organize their finances
   c. To help older adults plan for jobs after the age of 65
   d. To assist older adults in naming benefactors

71. Quality improvement (QI) refers to:
   a. Acute care and inpatient facilities only
   b. Attention to safety and appropriate care for all
   c. It has no importance to gerontological nursing.
   d. High-risk older adults only

72. Quality indicators for health-care research and patient safety appropriate for the older adult would include all of the following except:
   a. Wound care and decubitus ulcer prevention
   b. Postoperative hip fracture care
   c. Obstetric trauma
   d. Fall risk assessments

73. Which statement gives examples of educational programs for the older adult?
   a. Community programs that focus on lifestyle modifications
   b. Programs targeting specific age-related problems, such as nutrition, finances, or prevention
   c. Programs that focus on exercise for the older adult
   d. All of the above

74. The role of the gerontology nurse includes all of the following except:
   a. To facilitate the establishment of social support for the older adult
   b. To promote independent living as much as possible
   c. To educate and refer older adults to the appropriate resources
   d. All of the above

75. Which best describes what guides the appropriate nursing care of an aging adult?
   a. Evidence-based practice developed with ongoing research into the needs and outcomes of older adults
   b. General nursing care previously practiced
   c. Facility policies and procedures
   d. Physician orders for patient complaints

Answers and Explanations

1. D: It is important to understand how the client functions on a physical level with activities of daily living, but also on a psychological level by learning how the client copes, and a social level by assessing how the client functions within relationships.

2. A: Urinary incontinence is a common problem along with bladder leaking, frequency, and urinary tract infections. An in-depth assessment is needed to assist in diagnosing and treating urinary complaints in the older population. Exams should include history, physical examination of external genitalia, and pelvic or rectal exams.

3. B: The nurse must understand what is normal and what would be considered abnormal for the older adult patient when assessing for health needs. Although a basic understanding of financial difficulties, cardiac function, and sexual functioning is important, the nurse must differentiate the abnormal from the normal in order to help diagnose problems and improve outcomes for the patient.

4. C: It is the best initial question to ask a client over the age of 60 when assessing for cognitive function. While the other questions may be asked throughout the assessment, the client's perspective of memory and function is a baseline for the assessment. The client will usually be the first one to notice a change and is often too embarrassed or afraid to mention it to others.

5. B: Depression in those over the age of 65 is often under diagnosed and is directly related to the client's adjustment to this stage of ego integrity versus despair and how they view their life fulfillment.

6. A: An occasional lapse in memory is normal. Forgetting where you put your keys, forgetting that you have made an appointment, or forgetting to return a phone call can all be normal for busy adults. An adult over age 65 should still be able to recall the names of their children or siblings and their current address and be able to count to 10.

7. C: Depression and dementia are closely related to a decreased quality of life and functional decline. When a person loses functional abilities to do activities of daily living or activities that were once enjoyed, it can be viewed as having less of a full life, leading to depression and dementia.

8. A: There appears to be no change in the amount of medication absorbed other than with calcium due to the increase in gastric pH with aging. However, the rate of absorption appears to slow with aging, and adjustments in medication dosing may be altered to avoid toxicity.

9. C: Most age-related changes to drug absorption are linked to a decrease in body water and a decrease in lean body weight. Aging most often causes an increase in body fat and a decrease in serum albumin.

10. D: The liver is responsible for the majority of drug metabolism. Age-related decreases in liver blood flow may affect drug metabolism, as does liver pathology.

11. A: Doses of medications may need to be decreased when excreted primarily by the kidneys, especially in older adults or those with impaired renal function. Drugs such as morphine, which are metabolized in the liver but leave off by-products for excretion by the kidneys, may also need to be reduced in older adults.

12. A: ADRs are the result of overmedication, incorrect dosing, or incorrect managing of older adult medications. They put the client at risk for falls, cardiac problems, delirium, and many other side effects, leading to 16% of older adults needing hospitalization as a result. They increase the cost of health care, which exceeds billions of dollars each year just for ADRs.

13. B: Collagen and elastin are fibrous proteins in connective tissue that become stiff with age. Lipofuscin is a pigmented material that accumulates in aging tissue; cytoplasm shows changes with age, as does epithelial tissue.

14. C: Xerostomia, or dry mouth, is not a normal part of aging and is usually related to medications or medical conditions. It can affect nutrition, and assessment of oral hygiene and oral health should be performed to address this condition.

15. D: Vitamins for people over age 50 include increased vitamin D and additional vitamin B complex. Vitamins for those over 50 years of age have more iron and the recommended percentage of all nutrients, which the client may not be getting from healthy eating.

16. A: Is correct and was based on statistical analysis on mortality rates in the early 1900s. The other theories have been studied and researched more recently, when an increase of interest in the aging process and how to slow it down has gained popularity.

17. C: Neuroendocrine and immunological theories revolve around the idea that control of homeostasis and immune function can result in age-related changes. Answer a is part of molecular theory, answer b is part of evolutionary theory, and answer d is part of cellular theory.

18. D: There is a noticeable accumulation of lipofuscin in muscle and nervous tissue and an increase in lipids and fats in the tissue. There is a decrease in subcutaneous tissue, leading to an increase in wrinkles.

19. C: Organ tissue, thus the vital organs of the body, shows signs of decreasing function during the aging process. Although it takes place over a long period of time, stress and unexpected failures due to disease or trauma can hasten aging effects on the functional capacity of major organs.

20. B: Evidence-based practice offers a high potential for improving the health care provided to geriatric clients by the use of research findings and targeted results. Nurses play an important role in both research and practice in setting the standards for evidence-based practice in gerontological nursing.

21. C: Professionals trying to implement change into their practice use Rogers' diffusion of innovation model; it offers a systematic way to introduce changes for better outcomes in geriatric care. The other choices are incorrect.

22. B: Those clients over the age of 65 who have self-care needs that they cannot meet are appropriate for gerontological nursing care and may benefit from the services those nurses can provide. The other answers are completely false.

23. C: The gerontological nurse will use the nursing process and his or her advanced knowledge to assess and collect data from the aged client and his or her family. The nurse and the medical team use the data to develop diagnoses, which guide interventions. After assessing and deciding on the diagnosis, the nurse identifies expected outcomes, which focus on maximizing well-being. The nurse develops and implements a plan, including outside resources including education, prevention, rehabilitation, and palliative care. The nurse then continues to evaluate the plan and make changes to the interventions to work towards focused outcomes.

24. D: Gerontological nursing can be practiced wherever the client over the age of 65 seeks or receives health care. Health education can be provided at a community center as an outreach, care can be provided in the client's home, care can be initiated in an acute care setting when the client can no longer meet all of their own needs and an intervention may be needed, and it can be practiced in long-term care facilities. The role of the nurse in gerontology has expanded to reach clients through education, interventions, and as an advocate.

25. B: The nurse would do a complete history, physical, and assessment focusing on what the client feels he needs and how he feels his mind is functioning. The nurse most likely would speak to the family and, with the complete health-care team, develop a plan of action. The first reaction would not be to look for suitable nursing homes without first doing a full assessment and family/team conference.

26. C: When assessing the client's cognitive and perceptual patterns, the focus should be on changes in memory, difficulty in communicating or forming ideas, and orientation to time, place, and person. A client's perception of his or her financial status would not necessarily provide the nurse with concrete information with which to form a diagnosis and treatment plan.

27. D: It is normal for the nurse to ask about cardiac history in the aging adult due to the expectation that as you age you may experience cardiac problems, but we are not always comfortable asking about sexual history and expectations or if the older client is experiencing adult abuse. Both abuse and the topic of sexual activity should be part of a complete assessment to identify problems that may be occurring and could benefit from an intervention for overall well-being.

28. D: Theory not only identifies concepts but also offers the framework on which to base nursing practice interventions. The other choices are not correct, and answer a is not as completely correct as answer d.

29. B: Kolcaba's theory of comfort supports basic nursing care for the physical, psychosocial, and spiritual needs of the patient. Leininger and McFarland (2002) support the specialty of transcultural nursing with concepts on culture and health. Corbin and Strauss (1992) support the framework that describes the phases experienced with chronic illness and the responses to these phases. Norbeck, Lindsey, and Carrierei (1981) focus on the importance of social support to buffer life's stresses.

30. A: Older adults are more at risk for falls, especially when prescribed certain medications. These falls are a source for increased morbidity and death among those over 65. A fractured arm is not the most serious of all injuries that an older adult can experience. Depression is undertreated, and medications that treat depression should not necessarily be avoided just because the client is elderly.

31. B: Hyperglycemia may be an adverse reaction to the corticosteroids prescribed for the other three conditions.

32. A: If the patient is of sound mind and has been properly informed by a physician as to what DNR status means, the client is making a reasonable decision for herself. The other choices are not true.

33. B: Photoaging is the term used to describe the changes that skin develops as one ages. The other selections are not true.

34. C: Collagen is the substance that makes up the majority of the dermis. The other choices are all present in the dermis but at much smaller percentages of the total.

35. B: An aging adult may not be able to accept the cosmetic side of aging and opt for facelifts, Botox injections, and other cosmetic surgery in an attempt to look younger.

36. C: Senile purpura develops due to a loss of subcutaneous fat and connective tissue. The areas of discoloration occur on the hands and forearms where there is no protection for the capillaries, so any shearing or blunt force can cause bleeding under the skin. It can occur before the age of 60 depending on the medical condition of the client and is not related to an increase of blood vessels but more of a lack of protective padding over existing blood vessels. It is not usually related to medications.

37. C: Malignant melanoma is a highly malignant cancer that appears as pigmented areas. It spreads through the lymph system. Basal cell carcinoma, which arises from hair follicles, is the most common in Caucasian populations, but it is treatable and does not spread as easily. Squamous cell carcinoma is locally invasive and does not spread throughout the system. Actinic keratosis is associated with overexposure to the sun but is not malignant.

38. D: Is the most complete definition of the goals for treatment of leg ulcers in the elderly. Ulcers of the lower extremities develop due to venous stasis. The treatment then is not only to decrease the swelling, which promotes circulation, but also to eliminate infection, which promotes healing.

39. A: Bone softening and muscle weakness have the greatest effect on how the aging person can hold an erect position of standing, how he or she keeps a functional posture, and how he or she can continue to function on a daily basis. Weakness, fragility, posture, and degree of pain all affect daily functioning and independence. Nursing goals will be formed to help prevent further softening and muscle weakness and to promote independence.

40. B: The nurse realizes that aging effects on the musculoskeletal and nervous systems are slowing the movements of the elderly client and not necessarily cognitive function, laziness, or a recent medical change. It would be appropriate to assess the recent changes in relation to how the client can function, but the nurse realizes some degree of slowness is due to the effects of aging on muscles and bones.

41. C: While the other selections may be symptoms and need further evaluation, the nurse recognizes that they are not normal signs of aging. Resting tremors are normal for the aging adult, especially when he or she is extremely tired.

42. A: Paget's disease was first described by Sir James Paget in 1877. The effects of this disease over time can cause significant deformities and degenerative arthritis. The other selections are either not correct or they are fictitious.

43. B: These symptoms indicate osteoarthritis in the knee joint, and treatment recommendations and follow-up should be planned. Osteoporosis would not give a dry crackling sound and sensation nor would fluid in a joint. Although crepitation may be a normal symptom for someone previously diagnosed, it would not be considered a normal finding for someone initially complaining of knee pain.

44. C: Mild exercise and walking are suggested treatments for mild arthritis to help maintain mobility and function. Complete rest is recommended for a severe injury, as is ice. It is not the recommended treatment for coping with the disease on a daily basis.

45. A: These symptoms may be adverse reactions to the long-term salt therapy treatment with gold salts. The adverse reactions need to be weighed with the goals of treatment, and a new plan of therapy may need to be initiated.

46. C: NSAIDs can cause coagulation and bleeding problems, and education is important for those undergoing treatment with NSAIDs. These medications may also cause gastric irritation.

47. D: Hypertension, dyslipidemia, and diabetes all are contributing factors for CAD. While sexual orientation may indicate a need to evaluate for HIV/AIDS or other diseases, it is not a risk factor for CAD.

48. B: Studies show that lowering blood pressure in the older adult is the single most cost-effective way to prevent stroke, heart attacks, and ischemia. The other selections are either not as cost-effective for the older adult in preventing CAD, or they are incorrect.

49. C: Stage 1 hypertension guidelines include systolic pressures of 140 to 159 and diastolic pressures of 90 to 99. It is recommended to monitor the patient for six months if there is no history of hypertension and no present symptoms.

50. C: A patient may have complications from the CVA two months later, and physical complications and complaints would be the first order of business for the nurse to address. Financial concerns can be addressed at a later date with a case manager or social service professional after the initial physical recovery phase has begun.

51. A: Intermittent claudication is pain that is relieved by rest, extremities are usually cool, and pulses may be weak or absent.

52. A: The correct nursing diagnosis would be related to cardiac output. Answer b is incorrect because it would be an intolerance of activity. Answer c is incorrect because it should state decreases in cardiac output, and answer d is incorrect because the symptoms noted would not necessarily be for kidney failure.

53. D: Exercise most often will increase lung function in older adults.

54. A: You would not want to decrease exercise in a patient with COPD but rather slightly increase the patient's ability to tolerate some mild form of exercise or to improve exercise intolerance.

55. C: Although monitoring blood sugars may be part of daily routine labs, they most often do not indicate how a patient with pneumonia is responding. A blood sugar of 145 may be a normal finding depending on when the patient last ate.

56. A: Vertigo is a rotational sensation and is related to inner-ear disorders. Answer b refers to disequilibrium, answer c refers to syncope, and answer d refers to a presyncope symptom.

57. B: Patients who experience delirium should not be encouraged to ambulate and become excessively active before bed. The other choices are all appropriate nursing interventions.

58. C: Gastric biopsies, serum blood samples, and stool studies are all appropriate ways to diagnose H. pylori. The other choices would either be inappropriate or less effective treatments or diagnostic studies.

59. A: Older male clients with urinary complaints must be evaluated for prostate problems and hyperplasia. The other answers are incorrect.

60. C: Delayed arousal for older women can be a source of discouragement and lack of interest, as well as pain. A decrease in vaginal secretions may cause discomfort. A complete physical exam and open discussion with the client are needed to establish appropriate needs of the patient.

61. B: Bladder malignancies are common in the aging adult. The other choices may occur but are not related to the genitourinary system.

62. C: This drug is prescribed for incontinence and urgency when overflow is not the issue.

63. D: Kegel exercises are useful in stress incontinence but are generally not helpful with overflow incontinence. Methods to keep the bladder emptied are best suited for this symptom.

64. D: Constipation is most common with hyperthyroid disease.

65. B: Cataracts are the most common disease occurring in older adults requiring removal when vision is affected. Any of the other eye-related problems listed are not associated with the aging adult but can occur at any age.

66. D: The percentage of residents in a nursing home situation experiencing hearing loss is more than 70% and should be included in nursing care plans for those elderly residents but is often overlooked.

67. A: Aging adults most often experience a decrease in the ability to multitask.

68. D: This choice is not a delivery mode for reimbursement.

69. B: SSI refers to Supplemental Security Income. OAA refers to the Older American Act. Medicaid and Medicare were not designed to supplement Social Security.

70. A: This act encourages advance directives and patient choices with regards to end-of-life issues.

71. B: QI refers to safety and appropriate care regardless of the type of facility or the age of the client.

72. C: Obstetric trauma would not be something the older adult would encounter or be hospitalized for. In the rare occasion an older female would become pregnant, the facility may need to apply those patient standards, but, as a general rule, the older adult would not need safety standards for obstetric trauma to be in place.

73. D: All of the choices are examples of educational programs for the older adult. Hospital facilities often offer classes for older adults and support groups for older adults suffering with side effects from strokes, diabetes, muscle diseases, or grief.

74. D: All the selections encompass the role of the nurse caring for the older adult.

75. A: Gerontological nursing is based on years of clinical research and evidence-based practice guided by expected outcomes. The other selections do not offer a complete and holistic approach to care of the aging adult.

Secret Key #1 - Time is Your Greatest Enemy

Pace Yourself

Wear a watch. At the beginning of the test, check the time (or start a chronometer on your watch to count the minutes), and check the time after every few questions to make sure you are "on schedule."

If you are forced to speed up, do it efficiently. Usually one or more answer choices can be eliminated without too much difficulty. Above all, don't panic. Don't speed up and just begin guessing at random choices. By pacing yourself, and continually monitoring your progress against your watch, you will always know exactly how far ahead or behind you are with your available time. If you find that you are one minute behind on the test, don't skip one question without spending any time on it, just to catch back up. Take 15 fewer seconds on the next four questions, and after four questions you'll have caught back up. Once you catch back up, you can continue working each problem at your normal pace.

Furthermore, don't dwell on the problems that you were rushed on. If a problem was taking up too much time and you made a hurried guess, it must be difficult. The difficult questions are the ones you are most likely to miss anyway, so it isn't a big loss. It is better to end with more time than you need than to run out of time.

Lastly, sometimes it is beneficial to slow down if you are constantly getting ahead of time. You are always more likely to catch a careless mistake by working more slowly than quickly, and among very high-scoring test takers (those who are likely to have lots of time left over), careless errors affect the score more than mastery of material.

Secret Key #2 - Guessing is not Guesswork

You probably know that guessing is a good idea - unlike other standardized tests, there is no penalty for getting a wrong answer. Even if you have no idea about a question, you still have a 20-25% chance of getting it right.

Most test takers do not understand the impact that proper guessing can have on their score. Unless you score extremely high, guessing will significantly contribute to your final score.

Monkeys Take the Test

What most test takers don't realize is that to insure that 20-25% chance, you have to guess randomly. If you put 20 monkeys in a room to take this test, assuming they answered once per question and behaved themselves, on average they would get 20-25% of the questions correct. Put 20 test takers in the room, and the average will be much lower among guessed questions. Why?
  1. The test writers intentionally write deceptive answer choices that "look" right. A test taker has no idea about a question, so picks the "best looking" answer, which is often wrong. The

monkey has no idea what looks good and what doesn't, so will consistently be lucky about 20-25% of the time.

2. Test takers will eliminate answer choices from the guessing pool based on a hunch or intuition. Simple but correct answers often get excluded, leaving a 0% chance of being correct. The monkey has no clue, and often gets lucky with the best choice.

This is why the process of elimination endorsed by most test courses is flawed and detrimental to your performance- test takers don't guess, they make an ignorant stab in the dark that is usually worse than random.

$5 Challenge

Let me introduce one of the most valuable ideas of this course- the $5 challenge:

You only mark your "best guess" if you are willing to bet $5 on it.
You only eliminate choices from guessing if you are willing to bet $5 on it.

Why $5? Five dollars is an amount of money that is small yet not insignificant, and can really add up fast (20 questions could cost you $100). Likewise, each answer choice on one question of the test will have a small impact on your overall score, but it can really add up to a lot of points in the end.

The process of elimination IS valuable. The following shows your chance of guessing it right:

If you eliminate wrong answer choices until only this many remain:	Chance of getting it correct:
1	100%
2	50%
3	33%

However, if you accidentally eliminate the right answer or go on a hunch for an incorrect answer, your chances drop dramatically: to 0%. By guessing among all the answer choices, you are GUARANTEED to have a shot at the right answer.

That's why the $5 test is so valuable- if you give up the advantage and safety of a pure guess, it had better be worth the risk.
What we still haven't covered is how to be sure that whatever guess you make is truly random. Here's the easiest way:

Always pick the first answer choice among those remaining.

Such a technique means that you have decided, **before you see a single test question**, exactly how you are going to guess- and since the order of choices tells you nothing about which one is correct, this guessing technique is perfectly random.

This section is not meant to scare you away from making educated guesses or eliminating choices- you just need to define when a choice is worth eliminating. The $5 test, along with a pre-defined random guessing strategy, is the best way to make sure you reap all of the benefits of guessing.

Secret Key #3 - Practice Smarter, Not Harder

Many test takers delay the test preparation process because they dread the awful amounts of practice time they think necessary to succeed on the test. We have refined an effective method that will take you only a fraction of the time.

There are a number of "obstacles" in your way to succeed. Among these are answering questions, finishing in time, and mastering test-taking strategies. All must be executed on the day of the test at peak performance, or your score will suffer. The test is a mental marathon that has a large impact on your future.

Just like a marathon runner, it is important to work your way up to the full challenge. So first you just worry about questions, and then time, and finally strategy:

Success Strategy

1. Find a good source for practice tests.
2. If you are willing to make a larger time investment, consider using more than one study guide- often the different approaches of multiple authors will help you "get" difficult concepts.
3. Take a practice test with no time constraints, with all study helps "open book." Take your time with questions and focus on applying strategies.
4. ake a practice test with time constraints, with all guides "open book."
5. Take a final practice test with no open material and time limits

If you have time to take more practice tests, just repeat step 5. By gradually exposing yourself to the full rigors of the test environment, you will condition your mind to the stress of test day and maximize your success.

Secret Key #4 - Prepare, Don't Procrastinate

Let me state an obvious fact: if you take the test three times, you will get three different scores. This is due to the way you feel on test day, the level of preparedness you have, and, despite the test writers' claims to the contrary, some tests WILL be easier for you than others.

Since your future depends so much on your score, you should maximize your chances of success. In order to maximize the likelihood of success, you've got to prepare in advance. This means taking practice tests and spending time learning the information and test taking strategies you will need to succeed.

Never take the test as a "practice" test, expecting that you can just take it again if you need to. Feel free to take sample tests on your own, but when you go to take the official test, be prepared, be focused, and do your best the first time!

Secret Key #5 - Test Yourself

Everyone knows that time is money. There is no need to spend too much of your time or too little of your time preparing for the test. You should only spend as much of your precious time preparing as is necessary for you to get the score you need.

Once you have taken a practice test under real conditions of time constraints, then you will know if you are ready for the test or not.

If you have scored extremely high the first time that you take the practice test, then there is not much point in spending countless hours studying. You are already there.

Benchmark your abilities by retaking practice tests and seeing how much you have improved. Once you score high enough to guarantee success, then you are ready.

If you have scored well below where you need, then knuckle down and begin studying in earnest. Check your improvement regularly through the use of practice tests under real conditions. Above all, don't worry, panic, or give up. The key is perseverance!

Then, when you go to take the test, remain confident and remember how well you did on the practice tests. If you can score high enough on a practice test, then you can do the same on the real thing.

General Strategies

The most important thing you can do is to ignore your fears and jump into the test immediately- do not be overwhelmed by any strange-sounding terms. You have to jump into the test like jumping into a pool- all at once is the easiest way.

Make Predictions

As you read and understand the question, try to guess what the answer will be. Remember that several of the answer choices are wrong, and once you begin reading them, your mind will immediately become cluttered with answer choices designed to throw you off. Your mind is typically the most focused immediately after you have read the question and digested its contents. If you can, try to predict what the correct answer will be. You may be surprised at what you can predict.

Quickly scan the choices and see if your prediction is in the listed answer choices. If it is, then you can be quite confident that you have the right answer. It still won't hurt to check the other answer choices, but most of the time, you've got it!

Answer the Question

It may seem obvious to only pick answer choices that answer the question, but the test writers can create some excellent answer choices that are wrong. Don't pick an answer just because it sounds right, or you believe it to be true. It MUST answer the question. Once you've made your selection, always go back and check it against the question and make sure that you didn't misread the question, and the answer choice does answer the question posed.

Benchmark

After you read the first answer choice, decide if you think it sounds correct or not. If it doesn't, move on to the next answer choice. If it does, mentally mark that answer choice. This doesn't mean that you've definitely selected it as your answer choice, it just means that it's the best you've seen thus far. Go ahead and read the next choice. If the next choice is worse than the one you've already selected, keep going to the next answer choice. If the next choice is better than the choice you've already selected, mentally mark the new answer choice as your best guess.

The first answer choice that you select becomes your standard. Every other answer choice must be benchmarked against that standard. That choice is correct until proven otherwise by another answer choice beating it out. Once you've decided that no other answer choice seems as good, do one final check to ensure that your answer choice answers the question posed.

Valid Information

Don't discount any of the information provided in the question. Every piece of information may be necessary to determine the correct answer. None of the information in the question is there to throw you off (while the answer choices will certainly have information to throw you off). If two seemingly unrelated topics are discussed, don't ignore either. You can be confident there is a relationship, or it wouldn't be included in the question, and you are probably going to have to determine what is that relationship to find the answer.

Avoid "Fact Traps"

Don't get distracted by a choice that is factually true. Your search is for the answer that answers the question. Stay focused and don't fall for an answer that is true but incorrect. Always go back to the question and make sure you're choosing an answer that actually answers the question and is not just a true statement. An answer can be factually correct, but it MUST answer the question asked. Additionally, two answers can both be seemingly correct, so be sure to read all of the answer choices, and make sure that you get the one that BEST answers the question.

Milk the Question

Some of the questions may throw you completely off. They might deal with a subject you have not been exposed to, or one that you haven't reviewed in years. While your lack of knowledge about the subject will be a hindrance, the question itself can give you many clues that will help you find the correct answer. Read the question carefully and look for clues. Watch particularly for adjectives and nouns describing difficult terms or words that you don't recognize. Regardless of if you completely understand a word or not, replacing it with a synonym either provided or one you more familiar with may help you to understand what the questions are asking. Rather than wracking your mind about specific detailed information concerning a difficult term or word, try to use mental substitutes that are easier to understand.

The Trap of Familiarity

Don't just choose a word because you recognize it. On difficult questions, you may not recognize a number of words in the answer choices. The test writers don't put "make-believe" words on the test; so don't think that just because you only recognize all the words in one answer choice means that answer choice must be correct. If you only recognize words in one answer choice, then focus on that one. Is it correct? Try your best to determine if it is correct. If it is, that is great, but if it doesn't, eliminate it. Each word and answer choice you eliminate increases your chances of getting the question correct, even if you then have to guess among the unfamiliar choices.

Eliminate Answers

Eliminate choices as soon as you realize they are wrong. But be careful! Make sure you consider all of the possible answer choices. Just because one appears right, doesn't mean that the next one won't be even better! The test writers will usually put more than one good answer choice for every question, so read all of them. Don't worry if you are stuck between two that seem right. By getting down to just two remaining possible choices, your odds are now 50/50. Rather than wasting too much time, play the odds. You are guessing, but guessing wisely, because you've been able to knock out some of the answer choices that you know are wrong. If you are eliminating choices and realize that the last answer choice you are left with is also obviously wrong, don't panic. Start over and consider each choice again. There may easily be something that you missed the first time and will realize on the second pass.

Tough Questions

If you are stumped on a problem or it appears too hard or too difficult, don't waste time. Move on! Remember though, if you can quickly check for obviously incorrect answer choices, your chances of guessing correctly are greatly improved. Before you completely give up, at least try to knock out a couple of possible answers. Eliminate what you can and then guess at the remaining answer choices before moving on.

Brainstorm

If you get stuck on a difficult question, spend a few seconds quickly brainstorming. Run through the complete list of possible answer choices. Look at each choice and ask yourself, "Could this answer the question satisfactorily?" Go through each answer choice and consider it independently of the other. By systematically going through all possibilities, you may find something that you would otherwise overlook. Remember that when you get stuck, it's important to try to keep moving.

Read Carefully

Understand the problem. Read the question and answer choices carefully. Don't miss the question because you misread the terms. You have plenty of time to read each question thoroughly and make sure you understand what is being asked. Yet a happy medium must be attained, so don't waste too much time. You must read carefully, but efficiently.

Face Value

When in doubt, use common sense. Always accept the situation in the problem at face value. Don't read too much into it. These problems will not require you to make huge leaps of logic. The test writers aren't trying to throw you off with a cheap trick. If you have to go beyond creativity and make a leap of logic in order to have an answer choice answer the question, then you should look at the other answer choices. Don't overcomplicate the problem by creating theoretical relationships or explanations that will warp time or space. These are normal problems rooted in reality. It's just that the applicable relationship or explanation may not be readily apparent and you have to figure things out. Use your common sense to interpret anything that isn't clear.

Prefixes

If you're having trouble with a word in the question or answer choices, try dissecting it. Take advantage of every clue that the word might include. Prefixes and suffixes can be a huge help. Usually they allow you to determine a basic meaning. Pre- means before, post- means after, pro - is positive, de- is negative. From these prefixes and suffixes, you can get an idea of the general meaning of the word and try to put it into context. Beware though of any traps. Just because con is the opposite of pro, doesn't necessarily mean congress is the opposite of progress!

Hedge Phrases

Watch out for critical "hedge" phrases, such as likely, may, can, will often, sometimes, often, almost, mostly, usually, generally, rarely, sometimes. Question writers insert these hedge phrases to cover every possibility. Often an answer choice will be wrong simply because it leaves no room for exception. Avoid answer choices that have definitive words like "exactly," and "always".

Switchback Words

Stay alert for "switchbacks". These are the words and phrases frequently used to alert you to shifts in thought. The most common switchback word is "but". Others include although, however, nevertheless, on the other hand, even though, while, in spite of, despite, regardless of.

New Information

Correct answer choices will rarely have completely new information included. Answer choices typically are straightforward reflections of the material asked about and will directly relate to the question. If a new piece of information is included in an answer choice that doesn't even seem to relate to the topic being asked about, then that answer choice is likely incorrect. All of the information needed to answer the question is usually provided for you, and so you should not have to make guesses that are unsupported or choose answer choices that require unknown information that cannot be reasoned on its own.

Time Management

On technical questions, don't get lost on the technical terms. Don't spend too much time on any one question. If you don't know what a term means, then since you don't have a dictionary, odds are you aren't going to get much further. You should immediately recognize terms as whether or not you know them. If you don't, work with the other clues that you have, the other answer choices and terms provided, but don't waste too much time trying to figure out a difficult term.

Contextual Clues

Look for contextual clues. An answer can be right but not correct. The contextual clues will help you find the answer that is most right and is correct. Understand the context in which a phrase or statement is made. This will help you make important distinctions.

Don't Panic

Panicking will not answer any questions for you. Therefore, it isn't helpful. When you first see the question, if your mind goes blank, take a deep breath. Force yourself to mechanically go through the steps of solving the problem and using the strategies you've learned.

Pace Yourself

Don't get clock fever. It's easy to be overwhelmed when you're looking at a page full of questions, your mind is full of random thoughts and feeling confused, and the clock is ticking down faster than you would like. Calm down and maintain the pace that you have set for yourself. As long as you are on track by monitoring your pace, you are guaranteed to have enough time for yourself. When you get to the last few minutes of the test, it may seem like you won't have enough time left, but if you only have as many questions as you should have left at that point, then you're right on track!

Answer Selection

The best way to pick an answer choice is to eliminate all of those that are wrong, until only one is left and confirm that is the correct answer. Sometimes though, an answer choice may immediately look right. Be careful! Take a second to make sure that the other choices are not equally obvious. Don't make a hasty mistake. There are only two times that you should stop before checking other answers. First is when you are positive that the answer choice you have selected is correct. Second is when time is almost out and you have to make a quick guess!

Check Your Work

Since you will probably not know every term listed and the answer to every question, it is important that you get credit for the ones that you do know. Don't miss any questions through careless mistakes. If at all possible, try to take a second to look back over your answer selection and make sure you've selected the correct answer choice and haven't made a costly careless mistake (such as marking an answer choice that you didn't mean to mark). This quick double check should more than pay for itself in caught mistakes for the time it costs.

Beware of Directly Quoted Answers

Sometimes an answer choice will repeat word for word a portion of the question or reference section. However, beware of such exact duplication – it may be a trap! More than likely, the correct choice will paraphrase or summarize a point, rather than being exactly the same wording.

Slang

Scientific sounding answers are better than slang ones. An answer choice that begins "To compare the outcomes…" is much more likely to be correct than one that begins "Because some people insisted…"

Extreme Statements

Avoid wild answers that throw out highly controversial ideas that are proclaimed as established fact. An answer choice that states the "process should be used in certain situations, if…" is much more likely to be correct than one that states the "process should be discontinued completely." The first is a calm rational statement and doesn't even make a definitive, uncompromising stance, using a hedge word "if" to provide wiggle room, whereas the second choice is a radical idea and far more extreme.

Answer Choice Families

When you have two or more answer choices that are direct opposites or parallels, one of them is usually the correct answer. For instance, if one answer choice states "x increases" and another answer choice states "x decreases" or "y increases," then those two or three answer choices are very similar in construction and fall into the same family of answer choices. A family of answer choices is when two or three answer choices are very similar in construction, and yet often have a directly opposite meaning. Usually the correct answer choice will be in that family of answer choices. The "odd man out" or answer choice that doesn't seem to fit the parallel construction of the other answer choices is more likely to be incorrect.

Special Report: What Your Test Score Will Tell You About Your IQ

Did you know that most standardized tests correlate very strongly with IQ? In fact, your general intelligence is a better predictor of your success than any other factor, and most tests intentionally measure this trait to some degree to ensure that those selected by the test are truly qualified for the test's purposes.

Before we can delve into the relation between your test score and IQ, I will first have to explain what exactly is IQ. Here's the formula:

Your IQ = 100 + (Number of standard deviations below or above the average)*15

Now, let's define standard deviations by using an example. If we have 5 people with 5 different heights, then first we calculate the average. Let's say the average was 65 inches. The standard deviation is the "average distance" away from the average of each of the members. It is a direct measure of variability - if the 5 people included Jackie Chan and Shaquille O'Neal, obviously there's a lot more variability in that group than a group of 5 sisters who are all within 6 inches in height of each other. The standard deviation uses a number to characterize the average range of difference within a group.

A convenient feature of most groups is that they have a "normal" distribution- makes sense that most things would be normal, right? Without getting into a bunch of statistical mumbo-jumbo, you just need to know that if you know the average of the group and the standard deviation, you can successfully predict someone's percentile rank in the group.

Confused? Let me give you an example. If instead of 5 people's heights, we had 100 people, we could figure out their rank in height JUST by knowing the average, standard deviation, and their height. We wouldn't need to know each person's height and manually rank them, we could just predict their rank based on three numbers.

What this means is that you can take your PERCENTILE rank that is often given with your test and relate this to your RELATIVE IQ of people taking the test - that is, your IQ relative to the people taking the test. Obviously, there's no way to know your actual IQ because the people taking a standardized test are usually not very good samples of the general population- many of those with extremely low IQ's never achieve a level of success or competency necessary to complete a typical standardized test. In fact, professional psychologists who measure IQ actually have to use non-written tests that can fairly measure the IQ of those not able to complete a traditional test.

The bottom line is to not take your test score too seriously, but it is fun to compute your "relative IQ" among the people who took the test with you. I've done the calculations below. Just look up your percentile rank in the left and then you'll see your "relative IQ" for your test in the right hand column-

Percentile Rank	Your Relative IQ		Percentile Rank	Your Relative IQ
99	135		59	103
98	131		58	103
97	128		57	103
96	126		56	102
95	125		55	102
94	123		54	102
93	122		53	101
92	121		52	101
91	120		51	100
90	119		50	100
89	118		49	100
88	118		48	99
87	117		47	99
86	116		46	98
85	116		45	98
84	115		44	98
83	114		43	97
82	114		42	97
81	113		41	97
80	113		40	96
79	112		39	96
78	112		38	95
77	111		37	95
76	111		36	95
75	110		35	94
74	110		34	94
73	109		33	93
72	109		32	93
71	108		31	93
70	108		30	92
69	107		29	92
68	107		28	91
67	107		27	91
66	106		26	90
65	106		25	90
64	105		24	89
63	105		23	89
62	105		22	88
61	104		21	88
60	104		20	87

Special Report: What is Test Anxiety and How to Overcome It?

The very nature of tests caters to some level of anxiety, nervousness or tension, just as we feel for any important event that occurs in our lives. A little bit of anxiety or nervousness can be a good thing. It helps us with motivation, and makes achievement just that much sweeter. However, too much anxiety can be a problem; especially if it hinders our ability to function and perform.

"Test anxiety," is the term that refers to the emotional reactions that some test-takers experience when faced with a test or exam. Having a fear of testing and exams is based upon a rational fear, since the test-taker's performance can shape the course of an academic career. Nevertheless, experiencing excessive fear of examinations will only interfere with the test-takers ability to perform, and his/her chances to be successful.

There are a large variety of causes that can contribute to the development and sensation of test anxiety. These include, but are not limited to lack of performance and worrying about issues surrounding the test.

Lack of Preparation

Lack of preparation can be identified by the following behaviors or situations:

Not scheduling enough time to study, and therefore cramming the night before the test or exam
Managing time poorly, to create the sensation that there is not enough time to do everything
Failing to organize the text information in advance, so that the study material consists of the entire text and not simply the pertinent information
Poor overall studying habits

Worrying, on the other hand, can be related to both the test taker, or many other factors around him/her that will be affected by the results of the test. These include worrying about:

Previous performances on similar exams, or exams in general
How friends and other students are achieving
The negative consequences that will result from a poor grade or failure

There are three primary elements to test anxiety. Physical components, which involve the same typical bodily reactions as those to acute anxiety (to be discussed below). Emotional factors have to do with fear or panic. Mental or cognitive issues concerning attention spans and memory abilities.

Physical Signals

There are many different symptoms of test anxiety, and these are not limited to mental and emotional strain. Frequently there are a range of physical signals that will let a test taker know that he/she is suffering from test anxiety. These bodily changes can include the following:

Perspiring
Sweaty palms
Wet, trembling hands
Nausea
Dry mouth
A knot in the stomach
Headache
Faintness
Muscle tension
Aching shoulders, back and neck
Rapid heart beat
Feeling too hot/cold

To recognize the sensation of test anxiety, a test-taker should monitor him/herself for the following sensations:

The physical distress symptoms as listed above
Emotional sensitivity, expressing emotional feelings such as the need to cry or laugh too much, or a sensation of anger or helplessness
A decreased ability to think, causing the test-taker to blank out or have racing thoughts that are hard to organize or control.

Though most students will feel some level of anxiety when faced with a test or exam, the majority can cope with that anxiety and maintain it at a manageable level. However, those who cannot are faced with a very real and very serious condition, which can and should be controlled for the immeasurable benefit of this sufferer.

Naturally, these sensations lead to negative results for the testing experience. The most common effects of test anxiety have to do with nervousness and mental blocking.

Nervousness

Nervousness can appear in several different levels:

The test-taker's difficulty, or even inability to read and understand the questions on the test
The difficulty or inability to organize thoughts to a coherent form
The difficulty or inability to recall key words and concepts relating to the testing questions (especially essays)
The receipt of poor grades on a test, though the test material was well known by the test taker

Conversely, a person may also experience mental blocking, which involves:

Blanking out on test questions
Only remembering the correct answers to the questions when the test has already finished.

Fortunately for test anxiety sufferers, beating these feelings, to a large degree, has to do with proper preparation. When a test taker has a feeling of preparedness, then anxiety will be dramatically lessened.

The first step to resolving anxiety issues is to distinguish which of the two types of anxiety are being suffered. If the anxiety is a direct result of a lack of preparation, this should be considered a normal reaction, and the anxiety level (as opposed to the test results) shouldn't be anything to worry about. However, if, when adequately prepared, the test-taker still panics, blanks out, or seems to overreact, this is not a fully rational reaction. While this can be considered normal too, there are many ways to combat and overcome these effects.

Remember that anxiety cannot be entirely eliminated, however, there are ways to minimize it, to make the anxiety easier to manage. Preparation is one of the best ways to minimize test anxiety. Therefore the following techniques are wise in order to best fight off any anxiety that may want to build.

To begin with, try to avoid cramming before a test, whenever it is possible. By trying to memorize an entire term's worth of information in one day, you'll be shocking your system, and not giving yourself a very good chance to absorb the information. This is an easy path to anxiety, so for those who suffer from test anxiety, cramming should not even be considered an option.

Instead of cramming, work throughout the semester to combine all of the material which is presented throughout the semester, and work on it gradually as the course goes by, making sure to master the main concepts first, leaving minor details for a week or so before the test.

To study for the upcoming exam, be sure to pose questions that may be on the examination, to gauge the ability to answer them by integrating the ideas from your texts, notes and lectures, as well as any supplementary readings.

If it is truly impossible to cover all of the information that was covered in that particular term, concentrate on the most important portions, that can be covered very well. Learn these concepts as best as possible, so that when the test comes, a goal can be made to use these concepts as presentations of your knowledge.

In addition to study habits, changes in attitude are critical to beating a struggle with test anxiety. In fact, an improvement of the perspective over the entire test-taking experience can actually help a test taker to enjoy studying and therefore improve the overall experience. Be certain not to overemphasize the significance of the grade - know that the result of the test is neither a reflection of self worth, nor is it a measure of intelligence; one grade will not predict a person's future success.

To improve an overall testing outlook, the following steps should be tried:

Keeping in mind that the most reasonable expectation for taking a test is to expect to try to demonstrate as much of what you know as you possibly can.
Reminding ourselves that a test is only one test; this is not the only one, and there will be others. The thought of thinking of oneself in an irrational, all-or-nothing term should be avoided at all costs.
A reward should be designated for after the test, so there's something to look forward to. Whether it be going to a movie, going out to eat, or simply visiting friends, schedule it in advance, and do it no matter what result is expected on the exam.

Test-takers should also keep in mind that the basics are some of the most important things, even beyond anti-anxiety techniques and studying. Never neglect the basic social, emotional and biological needs, in order to try to absorb information. In order to best achieve, these three factors must be held as just as important as the studying itself.

Study Steps

Remember the following important steps for studying:

Maintain healthy nutrition and exercise habits. Continue both your recreational activities and social pass times. These both contribute to your physical and emotional well being.
Be certain to get a good amount of sleep, especially the night before the test, because when you're overtired you are not able to perform to the best of your best ability.
Keep the studying pace to a moderate level by taking breaks when they are needed, and varying the work whenever possible, to keep the mind fresh instead of getting bored.
When enough studying has been done that all the material that can be learned has been learned, and the test taker is prepared for the test, stop studying and do something relaxing such as listening to music, watching a movie, or taking a warm bubble bath.

There are also many other techniques to minimize the uneasiness or apprehension that is experienced along with test anxiety before, during, or even after the examination. In fact, there are a great deal of things that can be done to stop anxiety from interfering with lifestyle and performance. Again, remember that anxiety will not be eliminated entirely, and it shouldn't be. Otherwise that "up" feeling for exams would not exist, and most of us depend on that sensation to perform better than usual. However, this anxiety has to be at a level that is manageable.

Of course, as we have just discussed, being prepared for the exam is half the battle right away. Attending all classes, finding out what knowledge will be expected on the exam, and knowing the exam schedules are easy steps to lowering anxiety. Keeping up with work will remove the need to cram, and efficient study habits will eliminate wasted time. Studying should be done in an ideal location for concentration, so that it is simple to become interested in the material and give it complete attention. A method such as SQ3R (Survey, Question, Read, Recite, Review) is a wonderful key to follow to make sure that the study habits are as effective as possible, especially in the case of learning from a textbook. Flashcards are great techniques for memorization. Learning to take good notes will mean that notes will be full of useful information, so that less sifting will need to be done to seek out what is pertinent for studying. Reviewing notes after class and then again on occasion will keep the information fresh in the mind. From notes that have been taken summary sheets and outlines can be made for simpler reviewing.

A study group can also be a very motivational and helpful place to study, as there will be a sharing of ideas, all of the minds can work together, to make sure that everyone understands, and the studying will be made more interesting because it will be a social occasion.

Basically, though, as long as the test-taker remains organized and self confident, with efficient study habits, less time will need to be spent studying, and higher grades will be achieved.

To become self confident, there are many useful steps. The first of these is "self talk." It has been shown through extensive research, that self-talk for students who suffer from test anxiety, should be well monitored, in order to make sure that it contributes to self confidence as opposed to sinking the student. Frequently the self talk of test-anxious students is negative or self-defeating, thinking that everyone else is smarter and faster, that they always mess up, and that if they don't do well, they'll fail the entire course. It is important to decreasing anxiety that awareness is made of self talk. Try writing any negative self thoughts and then disputing them with a positive statement instead. Begin self-encouragement as though it was a friend speaking. Repeat positive statements to help reprogram the mind to believing in successes instead of failures.

Helpful Techniques

Other extremely helpful techniques include:

Self-visualization of doing well and reaching goals
While aiming for an "A" level of understanding, don't try to "overprotect" by setting your expectations lower. This will only convince the mind to stop studying in order to meet the lower expectations.
Don't make comparisons with the results or habits of other students. These are individual factors, and different things work for different people, causing different results.
Strive to become an expert in learning what works well, and what can be done in order to improve. Consider collecting this data in a journal.
Create rewards for after studying instead of doing things before studying that will only turn into avoidance behaviors.
Make a practice of relaxing - by using methods such as progressive relaxation, self-hypnosis, guided imagery, etc - in order to make relaxation an automatic sensation.

Work on creating a state of relaxed concentration so that concentrating will take on the focus of the mind, so that none will be wasted on worrying.
Take good care of the physical self by eating well and getting enough sleep.
Plan in time for exercise and stick to this plan.

Beyond these techniques, there are other methods to be used before, during and after the test that will help the test-taker perform well in addition to overcoming anxiety.

Before the exam comes the academic preparation. This involves establishing a study schedule and beginning at least one week before the actual date of the test. By doing this, the anxiety of not having enough time to study for the test will be automatically eliminated. Moreover, this will make the studying a much more effective experience, ensuring that the learning will be an easier process. This relieves much undue pressure on the test-taker.

Summary sheets, note cards, and flash cards with the main concepts and examples of these main concepts should be prepared in advance of the actual studying time. A topic should never be eliminated from this process. By omitting a topic because it isn't expected to be on the test is only setting up the test-taker for anxiety should it actually appear on the exam. Utilize the course syllabus for laying out the topics that should be studied. Carefully go over the notes that were made in class, paying special attention to any of the issues that the professor took special care to emphasize while lecturing in class. In the textbooks, use the chapter review, or if possible, the chapter tests, to begin your review.

It may even be possible to ask the instructor what information will be covered on the exam, or what the format of the exam will be (for example, multiple choice, essay, free form, true-false). Additionally, see if it is possible to find out how many questions will be on the test. If a review sheet or sample test has been offered by the professor, make good use of it, above anything else, for the preparation for the test. Another great resource for getting to know the examination is reviewing tests from previous semesters. Use these tests to review, and aim to achieve a 100% score on each of the possible topics. With a few exceptions, the goal that you set for yourself is the highest one that you will reach.

Take all of the questions that were assigned as homework, and rework them to any other possible course material. The more problems reworked, the more skill and confidence will form as a result. When forming the solution to a problem, write out each of the steps. Don't simply do head work. By doing as many steps on paper as possible, much clarification and therefore confidence will be formed. Do this with as many homework problems as possible, before checking the answers. By checking the answer after each problem, a reinforcement will exist, that will not be on the exam. Study situations should be as exam-like as possible, to prime the test-taker's system for the experience. By waiting to check the answers at the end, a psychological advantage will be formed, to decrease the stress factor.

Another fantastic reason for not cramming is the avoidance of confusion in concepts, especially when it comes to mathematics. 8-10 hours of study will become one hundred percent more effective if it is spread out over a week or at least several days, instead of doing it all in one sitting. Recognize that the human brain requires time in order to assimilate new material, so frequent breaks and a span of study time over several days will be much more beneficial.

Additionally, don't study right up until the point of the exam. Studying should stop a minimum of one hour before the exam begins. This allows the brain to rest and put things in their proper order. This will also provide the time to become as relaxed as possible when going into the examination room. The test-taker will also have time to eat well and eat sensibly. Know that the brain needs food as much as the rest of the body. With enough food and enough sleep, as well as a relaxed attitude, the body and the mind are primed for success.

Avoid any anxious classmates who are talking about the exam. These students only spread anxiety, and are not worth sharing the anxious sentimentalities.

Before the test also involves creating a positive attitude, so mental preparation should also be a point of concentration. There are many keys to creating a positive attitude. Should fears become rushing in, make a visualization of taking the exam, doing well, and seeing an A written on the paper. Write out a list of affirmations that will bring a feeling of confidence, such as "I am doing well in my English class," "I studied well and know my material," "I enjoy this class." Even if the affirmations aren't believed at first, it sends a positive message to the subconscious which will result in an alteration of the overall belief system, which is the system that creates reality.

If a sensation of panic begins, work with the fear and imagine the very worst! Work through the entire scenario of not passing the test, failing the entire course, and dropping out of school, followed by not getting a job, and pushing a shopping cart through the dark alley where you'll live. This will place things into perspective! Then, practice deep breathing and create a visualization of the opposite situation - achieving an "A" on the exam, passing the entire course, receiving the degree at a graduation ceremony.

On the day of the test, there are many things to be done to ensure the best results, as well as the most calm outlook. The following stages are suggested in order to maximize test-taking potential:

Begin the examination day with a moderate breakfast, and avoid any coffee or beverages with caffeine if the test taker is prone to jitters. Even people who are used to managing caffeine can feel jittery or light-headed when it is taken on a test day.
Attempt to do something that is relaxing before the examination begins. As last minute cramming clouds the mastering of overall concepts, it is better to use this time to create a calming outlook.
Be certain to arrive at the test location well in advance, in order to provide time to select a location that is away from doors, windows and other distractions, as well as giving enough time to relax before the test begins.
Keep away from anxiety generating classmates who will upset the sensation of stability and relaxation that is being attempted before the exam.
Should the waiting period before the exam begins cause anxiety, create a self-distraction by reading a light magazine or something else that is relaxing and simple.

During the exam itself, read the entire exam from beginning to end, and find out how much time should be allotted to each individual problem. Once writing the exam, should more time be taken for a problem, it should be abandoned, in order to begin another problem. If there is time at the end, the unfinished problem can always be returned to and completed.

Read the instructions very carefully - twice - so that unpleasant surprises won't follow during or after the exam has ended.

When writing the exam, pretend that the situation is actually simply the completion of homework within a library, or at home. This will assist in forming a relaxed atmosphere, and will allow the brain extra focus for the complex thinking function.

Begin the exam with all of the questions with which the most confidence is felt. This will build the confidence level regarding the entire exam and will begin a quality momentum. This will also create encouragement for trying the problems where uncertainty resides.

Going with the "gut instinct" is always the way to go when solving a problem. Second guessing should be avoided at all costs. Have confidence in the ability to do well.

For essay questions, create an outline in advance that will keep the mind organized and make certain that all of the points are remembered. For multiple choice, read every answer, even if the correct one has been spotted - a better one may exist.

Continue at a pace that is reasonable and not rushed, in order to be able to work carefully. Provide enough time to go over the answers at the end, to check for small errors that can be corrected.

Should a feeling of panic begin, breathe deeply, and think of the feeling of the body releasing sand through its pores. Visualize a calm, peaceful place, and include all of the sights, sounds and sensations of this image. Continue the deep breathing, and take a few minutes to continue this with closed eyes. When all is well again, return to the test.

If a "blanking" occurs for a certain question, skip it and move on to the next question. There will be time to return to the other question later. Get everything done that can be done, first, to guarantee all the grades that can be compiled, and to build all of the confidence possible. Then return to the weaker questions to build the marks from there.

Remember, one's own reality can be created, so as long as the belief is there, success will follow. And remember: anxiety can happen later, right now, there's an exam to be written!

After the examination is complete, whether there is a feeling for a good grade or a bad grade, don't dwell on the exam, and be certain to follow through on the reward that was promised...and enjoy it! Don't dwell on any mistakes that have been made, as there is nothing that can be done at this point anyway.

Additionally, don't begin to study for the next test right away. Do something relaxing for a while, and let the mind relax and prepare itself to begin absorbing information again.

From the results of the exam - both the grade and the entire experience, be certain to learn from what has gone on. Perfect studying habits and work some more on confidence in order to make the next examination experience even better than the last one.

Learn to avoid places where openings occurred for laziness, procrastination and day dreaming.

Use the time between this exam and the next one to better learn to relax, even learning to relax on cue, so that any anxiety can be controlled during the next exam. Learn how to relax the body. Slouch in your chair if that helps. Tighten and then relax all of the different muscle groups, one group at a time, beginning with the feet and then working all the way up to the neck and face. This will ultimately relax the muscles more than they were to begin with. Learn how to breathe deeply and comfortably, and focus on this breathing going in and out as a relaxing thought. With every exhale, repeat the word "relax."

As common as test anxiety is, it is very possible to overcome it. Make yourself one of the test-takers who overcome this frustrating hindrance.

Special Report: Retaking the Test: What Are Your Chances at Improving Your Score?

After going through the experience of taking a major test, many test takers feel that once is enough. The test usually comes during a period of transition in the test taker's life, and taking the test is only one of a series of important events. With so many distractions and conflicting recommendations, it may be difficult for a test taker to rationally determine whether or not he should retake the test after viewing his scores.

The importance of the test usually only adds to the burden of the retake decision. However, don't be swayed by emotion. There a few simple questions that you can ask yourself to guide you as you try to determine whether a retake would improve your score:

1. What went wrong? Why wasn't your score what you expected?

Can you point to a single factor or problem that you feel caused the low score? Were you sick on test day? Was there an emotional upheaval in your life that caused a distraction? Were you late for the test or not able to use the full time allotment? If you can point to any of these specific, individual problems, then a retake should definitely be considered.

2. Is there enough time to improve?

Many problems that may show up in your score report may take a lot of time for improvement. A deficiency in a particular math skill may require weeks or months of tutoring and studying to improve. If you have enough time to improve an identified weakness, then a retake should definitely be considered.

3. How will additional scores be used? Will a score average, highest score, or most recent score be used?

Different test scores may be handled completely differently. If you've taken the test multiple times, sometimes your highest score is used, sometimes your average score is computed and used, and sometimes your most recent score is used. Make sure you understand what method will be used to evaluate your scores, and use that to help you determine whether a retake should be considered.

4. Are my practice test scores significantly higher than my actual test score?

If you have taken a lot of practice tests and are consistently scoring at a much higher level than your actual test score, then you should consider a retake. However, if you've taken five practice tests and only one of your scores was higher than your actual test score, or if your practice test scores were only slightly higher than your actual test score, then it is unlikely that you will significantly increase your score.

5. Do I need perfect scores or will I be able to live with this score? Will this score still allow me to follow my dreams?

What kind of score is acceptable to you? Is your current score "good enough?" Do you have to have a certain score in order to pursue the future of your dreams? If you won't be happy with your current score, and there's no way that you could live with it, then you should consider a retake. However, don't get your hopes up. If you are looking for significant improvement, that may or may not be possible. But if you won't be happy otherwise, it is at least worth the effort. Remember that there are other considerations. To achieve your dream, it is likely that your grades may also be taken into account. A great test score is usually not the only thing necessary to succeed. Make sure that you aren't overemphasizing the importance of a high test score.

Furthermore, a retake does not always result in a higher score. Some test takers will score lower on a retake, rather than higher. One study shows that one-fourth of test takers will achieve a significant improvement in test score, while one-sixth of test takers will actually show a decrease. While this shows that most test takers will improve, the majority will only improve their scores a little and a retake may not be worth the test taker's effort.

Finally, if a test is taken only once and is considered in the added context of good grades on the part of a test taker, the person reviewing the grades and scores may be tempted to assume that the test taker just had a bad day while taking the test, and may discount the low test score in favor of the high grades. But if the test is retaken and the scores are approximately the same, then the validity of the low scores are only confirmed. Therefore, a retake could actually hurt a test taker by definitely bracketing a test taker's score ability to a limited range.

Special Report: Additional Bonus Material

Due to our efforts to try to keep this book to a manageable length, we've created a link that will give you access to all of your additional bonus material.

Please visit http://www.mometrix.com/bonus948/cnsgeron to access the information.